THE 5 Resets

THE 5 Resets

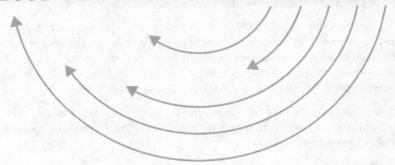

Rewire Your Brain and Body for Less Stress and More Resilience

ADITI NERURKAR, MD

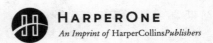

HarperOne
An Imprint of HarperCollins*Publishers*

These narratives have been written to reflect common patterns and themes I've seen in my clinical practice over the past two decades and in my interactions with thousands of patients. No actual person is represented by them or by the names or clinical conditions used. Any similarity to an actual person or a conversation with an actual person is a reflection of these frequent patient concerns. Quotations are paraphrased so as to convey my overall breadth of experience.

The content of this book is provided for informational purposes and does not establish a doctor-patient relationship. It may not be used for diagnosis and is not a substitute for advice, diagnosis, or treatment with a licensed physician or mental healthcare professional. The author and publisher do not assume responsibility for how the reader may choose to apply the information provided.

References do not constitute an endorsement of any author, book, website, or other source material. Websites may change over time.

HarperCollins books may be purchased for educational, business, or sales promotional use. For information, please email the Special Markets Department at SPsales@harpercollins.com.

FIRST EDITION

Designed by Janet Evans-Scanlon
Illustrations © pixssa/Shutterstock

Library of Congress Cataloging-in-Publication Data has been applied for.

ISBN 978-0-06-328921-5

23 24 25 26 27 LBC 5 4 3 2 1

To Mac and Zoë, my resets

Contents

THE 5 Resets

Introduction

One night in May, I got a call from my invincible longtime friend Liz. She was in a panic.

"I'm not sure what's going on with me," she confided. "I've completely lost my motivation to work out."

Now for most of us, a resistance to exercise is everyday life, but for my friend Liz it was a true reckoning. Since the first day I met her, more than twenty-five years ago, she's jumped out of bed every day at 5:30 a.m. to exercise. She's run ultramarathons, done Ironmans, and climbed literal mountains. She exercised her way through graduate school, a twelve-year marriage, and two pregnancies. She's like a Marvel Comics superhero. Liz's superpower has always been her insane physical prowess. So when she called me that night saying she hadn't exercised in six months, my antenna went up.

"It's not like I lie on the couch all day and mope," Liz told me. "So it's definitely not burnout. You know me. I'm resilient."

I stayed quiet and listened, but as a Harvard-trained doctor with an expertise in stress and burnout, I recognized what I call the resilience myth—the idea that putting your head down and powering through rough times is what resilience is all about (see Chapter 1). I could hear the familiar voice of the resilience myth when Liz said, "I'm working constantly. My mind never shuts off. But I can't shake the feeling of being really depleted. Every morning, I hit snooze on my alarm and don't exercise at all."

She sounded more exhausted than I'd ever heard her.

"What do you think is going on?" she asked.

My diagnosis was pretty clear. "You have chronic stress and atypical burnout," I told her.

Of course, she didn't believe me right away. It took another twenty minutes of my relaying the hard scientific data on stress and then having her answer some questions I often ask my patients so they can score their stress level, from 1 (low) to 20 (high); see Chapter 1.

Despite her history of invincibility, Liz's stress was definitely in the high range. Together, her three symptoms—an inability to unplug from work, feeling depleted, and a stark change from her usual exercise habit—pointed to the picture of chronic stress and burnout. By the end of our conversation, she was convinced.

"How do I fix this?" Liz asked me. "Nothing I'm doing is working."

My suggestion was a regimen of some simple and actionable lifestyle changes, beginning with only two changes at a time. These changes were practical and easy enough for her to incorporate into an already overscheduled life. She could start them that same day.

Three months later, Liz was on her way back to bouncing out of bed at 5:30 a.m. for a five-mile run, and she's never looked back.

In this book, you'll find out how and why each of my simple research-backed techniques helped my friend Liz and how they can help you, too. In these current times, stress and burnout aren't the exception, they're the rule. In several nationwide surveys people said that the past few years have been the most stressful time of their entire professional lives,[1] and more than 75 percent of adults have experienced burnout.[2]

Stress and burnout are two of the biggest and most universal issues plaguing our modern world. The good news is that they're both fully reversible and can be overcome by using the small, actionable techniques described in this book. Using the techniques, mixed with a healthy dose of self-compassion, you can overcome your stress and burnout in about three months.

This isn't about the latest fad, fix, or hack to improve overnight. Your brain and body are too smart for hacks; they see right through them. This book offers sustainable, far-reaching, and long-lasting changes, along with a couple of powerful mindset shifts, that can teach you how to reverse your biology of stress for good.

Contrary to what you may have been told, stress isn't a sign that you're weak at handling the demands of everyday life or that you've failed as a human being. Stress is a normal part of the human experience. I mean, if my invincible friend who seems to be part of the Marvel Universe could feel the impact of stress, then so can you.

You've been misled by modern society and our current hustle culture that stress is a sign of weakness, an embarrassment, something to cover up and hide at all costs. But stress isn't the enemy; our cultural perception of it is. Allow me to debunk all of these negative notions about stress for you.

As a doctor, I've dedicated myself to specializing in the biology of stress, burnout, mental health, and resilience. I've done a deep dive into what stress is and how it can and often does become unhealthy for each of us at one time or another. I've uncovered why it goes undiagnosed and how the current treatments only offer temporary fixes, not long-term solutions for any of us.

Here's the secret that the multibillion-dollar wellness industry doesn't want you to know: life without stress is biologically impossible. Forget those false promises you might have read or seen that tell you that you can magically get rid of stress forever if you take this or try that product. That's false advertising!

Stress is one of life's great paradoxes. It's the most common experience we can have as humans. But instead of unifying us, it isolates us, making us feel alone in our struggle. While running a stress-management clinic in Boston, I saw this play out every day, one patient at a time. But when I was invited to speak to large international audiences about my findings on unhealthy stress and my science-backed techniques to reset it, I fully grasped the vastness of the stress paradox.

I've had the opportunity to communicate with tens of thousands of people from all walks of life about the impact of unhealthy stress and burnout on mental and physical health. No matter where in the world I've shared my work about stress with people, I've found one very astonishing similarity. Regardless of their country, age, or occupation, each person's stress concerns were almost identical. Whether a factory line worker in Asia, a CEO in Europe, a tech programmer in Silicon Valley, or a childcare provider in North America, the one thing they all had in common was how they defined their concerns with stress. They grappled with the demands of their roles at work; their commitments as parents, caregivers, and partners; and most of all, how the shifting expectations of their daily lives affected their mental and physical health. In my experience, these patterns have been remarkably similar across a variety of cultures, sometimes down to the precise wording of the questions I'm asked about overcoming an individual's stress experience.

We may each have a personal stress story, but after conversations with thousands of people all around the world, I've uncovered and summarized five universal truths regarding stress. Chances are, if you've struggled with your stress these past few years, then you've experienced at least one—but very likely all five—of these universal concerns.

1. I feel anxious when faced with uncertainty, and I struggle to control my emotions during difficult experiences.

2. I don't feel rested in mind or body and spend most days feeling depleted.

3. I have so much stress that I accomplish very little, yet at the same time, I feel too burned out to be productive.

4. I have so many roles to fill between work, family, and community that I have little sense of myself anymore.

5. I don't find any purpose and meaning to my life while I face so many personal or professional struggles.

If one or more of these five concerns resonates with you, it may seem like your life has been taken over by stress.

The truth is, stress is a natural part of your life, as much as feeling hunger or needing to sleep. Stress is in fact an important default pathway in your brain. It's deeply tied to your lived experience and so essential to being human that it's the very foundation on which your brain, body, and biology are built. Stress isn't the enemy. It's what makes you, you. It's the driving force that gets you up out of bed every morning and propels you forward throughout the day.

Chances are, everything good in your life was created because of a little bit of stress. You graduated and got your first job as a result of healthy stress. It helped you start a new friendship with your current best friend. When you're rooting for your favorite sports team every season, a little healthy stress is involved. It has even helped you take your favorite vacation and plan for the next one. Healthy stress has had a guiding hand throughout your life in big and small ways.

A healthy amount of stress is important because it's an adaptive response to life's many demands. It serves a functional purpose to move your life forward, but only when it's dialed to the right frequency for you. The key is to figure out just how much stress is too much stress for you.

Stress becomes unhealthy when it's dysfunctional and out of tune with the frequency of your life. When stress starts having a life of its own and becomes a runaway train, that's when it gets difficult to manage and contain. This type of runaway stress no longer serves a beneficial purpose in your life. It becomes counterproductive and can end up being harmful to your health and well-being.

My goal is to help you reset your stress, learn how to manage it using healthy boundaries, and eventually master the skills and techniques needed to decrease your unhealthy stress so it doesn't consume every aspect of your life. You can't erase all of your stress forever, but you can get rid of the dysfunctional, unhealthy stress in your life that keeps you feeling depleted and burned out.

The 5 Resets in this book, which I've developed through my extensive experience in helping people understand and reduce stress, will teach you how to pump the brakes and slow down your runaway, counterproductive stress and reset your brain and body so that stress can serve you, not hurt you. What does it mean to reset your stress? A reset clears any pending errors and brings a system back into optimal condition. As you already know, you can reset a stopwatch, a broken bone, or a computer. This book contains insights, techniques, and principles for how to reset your stress.

Within each of The 5 Resets you'll find information and easy-to-apply tools that are backed by scientific research and have a proven track record with patients in my professional life, whose stories will illustrate the why and the how of each technique. You'll find out how to rewire your brain and body for less stress and more resilience from the inside out through incremental changes over time. The 5 Resets are:

1. **Get Clear on What Matters Most.** This reset will get your head in the game by cultivating the right mindset to rewire your brain and body.

2. **Find Quiet in a Noisy World.** You'll learn techniques on how to protect your mental bandwidth by minimizing external influences.

3. **Sync Your Brain and Your Body.** With this reset, you will focus on simple and effective techniques to help your brain and body serve you better during periods of high stress.

4. **Come Up for Air.** You'll learn practical and actionable techniques to cement your newfound wisdom into the constraints of everyday life.

5. **Bring Your Best Self Forward.** This reset will teach you a powerful new language for your brain and body to redefine your relationship to stress.

Within The 5 Resets, you'll discover clearly defined and manageable ways to work with your biology, rather than against it, through fifteen specific, research-backed techniques that will help you rewire your brain and body for a whole new level of resilience and far fewer negative effects of unhealthy stress, day by day. How can I be so sure? Because I've had the honor of witnessing thousands of patient transformations, and I want you to join the success stories I share in this book.

Perhaps like me, your privacy is important to you. I want you to know that every technique I include in this book can be done privately in your own home, or silently, without anyone around you even knowing you're practicing a technique to manage your stress or burnout. You won't need to do anything special, such as set aside extra time, join a gym, or purchase equipment. The techniques are free and simple and will not draw any unwanted attention to your practicing stress management in your professional or personal life. Everything you'll read in The 5 Resets has one purpose: to help you make huge strides in managing your stress and burnout, cultivating the right kind of resilience and fostering a deep sense of health and well-being.

From combating the burnout of work and parenting, managing the grief of losing someone dear, or the overwhelm that comes from having a new medical condition, I've helped many people over the past twenty years navigate the most challenging times in their lives and taught them how to recover and rebuild themselves from the inside out. Unquestionably, we've lived through uncertain and rapidly changing times in the past few years, which have taken a huge toll on our mental and physical health. We've faced their harsh repercussions on ourselves, our loved ones, our workplaces, our schools, and nearly every aspect of our daily lives, not to mention the overall economy and state of the world. But even if you feel like your life is in shambles, my deepest belief is that you have all the tools within yourself to rise up, meet the challenge of the moment, and become stronger than ever. Your time is now, and I'm going to help you by offering easy guidance that you can follow every step of the way.

I'll walk with you through each of The 5 Resets so you arrive at your destination with a clear understanding of how stress impacts your brain and body and, most importantly, what you can do to feel better, calmer, and more empowered to take control of your life again. Each technique is a simple, practical, and action-oriented tool to help you outsmart your biology, reset your stress, and supercharge your resilience. I've applied all of these techniques to my own life during my personal stress story. I know the benefits they've had for me and how they've also helped the many patients I've cared for over the years. My own journey as a doctor, researcher, and patient (we'll get to that in Chapter 1) has shown me that at the center of every human story is a theme of resilience. I've seen this play out hundreds of times with my patients, and I know there's a story of resilience within you.

Through my nearly two decades of training, clinical work, and research, I've had the great privilege of observing the inner workings of human beings up close. I'm the keeper of so many stories that began with stress and pain but ended in perseverance and triumph. If you've picked up this book, you've already taken the first most important step to less stress and more resilience. You may have spent many days feeling stressed, burned out, and completely depleted. You may be wondering whether you'll ever get through the dark tunnel of stress and return to a life where you feel more in control and have a better frame of mind. You may not believe me, but I promise that if you follow through with The 5 Resets, your story of resilience is the one you'll be telling. Just like my friend Liz the superhero, you have the superpower of resilience that's just waiting to emerge, and I'm going to help you discover it.

1

What's Your Stress Really Telling You?

I was dripping with sweat even though I was standing still. I was dizzy. Inside my chest, I felt something new, different, and terrifying. A stampede of wild horses. The air was being knocked out of me. I had a hard time catching my breath.

I was in the cardiac intensive care unit in a city called "the most dangerous city in America" in 2007. But I wasn't a patient; I was the doctor. At that moment, I was calmly and methodically making my patient rounds, something I'd done every day for the previous two years.

I was the doctor in charge and fully in control, but in my body, things felt out of control. I was at a standstill in the doorway of a patient's room, trying hard to stop whatever was happening inside me, quite seriously wondering whether I should be the patient in that hospital room instead.

The nurse I was working with immediately sensed something wasn't right. She told me to sit down and brought me some orange juice to drink. Seconds later, the feeling passed, and we both laughed it off. "It's probably just low blood sugar from working overnight and not eating enough," she said.

I'd been on call the night before, and we'd had many hospital admissions. I'd had no time to eat a full meal, stay hydrated, or even use the bathroom—common occurrences for doctors in training. But still, something else seemed off, and the sensation had me shaking in my scrubs, literally. What had just happened to me?

I'd been working eighty hours a week in my medical training for the previous few years, spending every third night in the hospital on overnight call. It was a coveted training program for the real-world exposure we received, an ideal learning environment for young doctors like me. But the unpredictable and harsh reality for doctors in training could be intense and sometimes shocking. One night, I saw a pregnant woman being wheeled on a gurney into the trauma ER with bullet wounds in her abdomen. We saw some gruesome stuff, but there wasn't a spare moment to pause, catch our breath, or process what we witnessed. We simply kept going. There was always another seriously ill patient who needed our attention.

If I had a few minutes to spare in the hospital, I'd grab a cold turkey sandwich and a supersize caffeinated drink from the cafeteria and eat on my feet while making notes in patient charts. I rarely saw sunshine, except through the hospital windows. I didn't exercise unless you count running from one patient room to the next. My sleep was erratic, at best. If things were quiet on overnight calls, I would catch a couple hours of rest in the doctor-on-call room on a worn-out bunk bed. On busy nights, I didn't.

It's how the medical trainee world worked at that time. There was no spare moment to process anything, good or bad. We didn't have the right terminology to describe the emotional aspects of our medical trainee experience. The words "self-care," "stress," and "burnout" didn't exist in my vocabulary nor anyone else's two decades ago in the clinical world.

I never questioned any of it because I wanted to be counted as someone who could handle it all, like I had been taught to do.

Many years before I felt those wild horses in my chest, a teacher at medical school had told me, "Pressure makes diamonds, Aditi. By the end of medical training, you're all going to be gleaming diamonds."

I believed him. I became strongly rooted in that belief. I loved the thrilling intensity of my work, so I unknowingly bought in to the resilience myth (see below) and persevered through every stage of my trainee experience because, hey . . . diamond in the making here.

But my body told a different story.

That day in the cardiac ICU was the first and last time I ever felt those wild horses during my waking hours. Instead, the palpitations followed me home and visited my body at night just as I was relaxed enough to fall asleep. I'd be jolted awake by the scary, out-of-the blue sensations. After a half hour or more, I'd drift off to sleep, exhausted and in need of rest. Of course, I was terrified. But I kept it to myself. I thought it was a passing phase. I'd heard about medical student syndrome, a phenomenon where you feel your patients' symptoms. Since I was the doctor in the cardiac ICU taking care of people's hearts, maybe I had just become more aware of my own?

What I didn't know then that I do know now is that my bedtime-only palpitations were a classic manifestation of the delayed stress response. When we're stressed, our brains have an uncanny ability to rise up and meet the moment by compartmentalizing inconvenient aspects of ourselves that don't help with our immediate self-preservation. But after the acute stressful experience has passed and things have settled down, like at bedtime, our true emotions come to the surface. It's something I've seen and recognized in my own patients and thousands of other people over the past twenty years. But when it first happened to me, nothing made sense. My palpitations continued for weeks, every single night, just as I lay my head down to sleep. Once my rotation in the cardiac ICU was finished, I thought it would all resolve. But it didn't. It continued on, night after frustrating night.

Completely fed up with this unsolvable issue, I finally hit my limit and went to see a doctor. I wanted to find a solution quickly and get back to my life as it had been before the nightly stampede. I was perplexed because even though I knew about the physiology of the body, I still couldn't figure out what was happening to me. I decided to cut to the chase and have a full workup. I had blood tests for electrolytes and infection, thyroid hormone levels, and anemia markers; multiple blood pressure and heart rate checks; an electrocardiogram; and even a heart ultrasound. My results came in.

The doctor smiled enthusiastically. "Everything looks great. It's all within normal limits."

She was happy. I was confused.

"Maybe it's stress?" she said reassuringly, as she ushered me out the door. "Try to relax when you can. I know it's hard with medical training. I've been there."

I wasn't reassured at all.

It seemed impossible that the very real symptoms I was feeling could be due to stress. Seriously, how could something so benign like stress affect me physically with such force and intensity? It didn't make sense. I'd already gone through so many stressful experiences in my medical training, why would stress suddenly affect me now? Stress didn't happen to resilient people like me! I thought I'd be immune to the harmful effects of stress. I had a reputation for an incomparable work ethic, and I wore that label proudly like a medal of honor. There's no way that stress had backed me into a corner. I left the doctor's office in disbelief and with no real solutions to my struggle.

Not seeing any other options, however, I took the doctor's advice and found ways to relax more. Whenever I had a rare day off, I watched movies, spent time with family and friends, went shopping, and even tried a spa. It didn't change anything. Every night, the stampede came back at bedtime.

Relaxing more wasn't working. I didn't need a distraction; I needed answers. After one particularly grueling thirty-hour work shift at the hospital, I walked past a yoga studio in my neighborhood. On a whim, I went in and took my first yoga class. I was still wearing my hospital scrubs. I stretched and twisted myself into poses that were strange to me. I learned some new breathing techniques.

That night, I slept more soundly than I had in weeks. The horses still showed up, but they were less intense and left more quickly. Could a yoga class have that effect or was it a coincidence? I had to know. I decided to test my hypothesis and began taking yoga classes twice a week. My teacher also gave us some breathing exercises to do at home. They were simple techniques that I could integrate into my daily life without having to shift my whole schedule. I also started walking to and from work. I drank less caffeine during the day and went to bed earlier whenever I could. If I wasn't on call, I began silencing my phone at bedtime.

Even though I had no scientific proof that any of this was helping me, I slowly started to feel better. My wild mustang stampede every night slowly became more like a trot of circus ponies across my chest.

For the next three months, even while working eighty hours per week, I committed to a plan of daily walks, an early bedtime, less caffeine, and yoga and breathing exercises. My palpitations diminished little by little, and one night they disappeared completely, never to be experienced again. That was almost twenty years ago. They've never come back. And I can't say I miss them.

I found my way back through the dark tunnel of stress by testing techniques that were new to me, making lifestyle choices that transformed my body's response to stress by tapping into the *mind-body connection*—the idea that our thoughts and feelings can directly affect our bodies in both positive and negative ways (see Chapter 5). Because I had this new experience, I wanted to do everything in my power to protect my mindset.

Eventually, the scientist part of my brain kicked in. What the hell had happened to me with stress, and how had I found my way to the other side? I wanted to uncover the scientific rationale behind my experience. I dug deeply and researched extensively, reading everything I could on the biology of stress. Like Alice in Wonderland, I entered a new and vibrant world that was outside of my conventional medical training. How is it that stress, the most common phenomenon to happen to nearly every human on the planet, wasn't something we talked about or offered real solutions for in a doctor's office?

I knew what I had to do next. I wanted to become the doctor I desperately had needed and hadn't been able to find when I suffered from my stress experience. I wanted to be the one to give stressed people, like me, tangible and scientific tools they could use in their busy everyday lives to transform their own stress, the same way I had done for myself.

So that's what I did.

I applied for and was accepted into a clinical research fellowship at Harvard Medical School where I studied the biology of stress and the mind-body connection. In my research, I uncovered the startling finding that even though 60 percent to 80 percent of visits to a doctor have a stress-related component, only 3 percent of doctors counsel their patients on stress management.[1] My personal experience with my own doctor lined up with this research. I bet it has for you, too.

You might be wondering why, if stress is such a common culprit for physical symptoms and medical issues, it has been so ignored by conventional Western medicine? Why doesn't your doctor talk about stress as the reason you're not sleeping through the night? Or when you tell your doctor you feel queasy every Sunday when spending time with your in-laws, why hasn't he or she ever brought up stress? Is the neck pain that happens every Tuesday morning during your weekly team meeting at your job caused by stress?

Stress is today's buzzword—we see it everywhere in the news and on social media—but when it comes to linking the negative effects of runaway stress with our medical symptoms, there's a gap. Stress still lives in the shadows of the conventional Western medical system and hasn't taken center stage, despite it being ever-present in nearly all doctors' visits.

Whenever someone asks me what my specialty is, I say, "I talk to patients about the elephant in the exam room—their stress. I also address the emotional component of chronic illness and serve as a bridge between high tech and high touch."

So much of clinical medicine involves the latest high-tech treatment. It's what makes our conventional medical system one of the best in the world. I'm a huge proponent of that system when it comes to acute, life-threatening conditions because it saves millions of lives. But along with our emphasis on the many high-tech interventions, we need to equally value the high-touch aspects of medical care that have been far too neglected. Doctors need to make patients feel like people first and conditions second, to help them feel seen, heard and understood for their lived experience, which is difficult for us to do well in our current medical system.

This isn't about the failings of individual physicians. Doctors find ways to move mountains every day for their patients, despite the larger systemic forces at play that get in the way of doing their jobs.

It's never about an individual; it's about a broken system. Most doctors would wholeheartedly agree.

Thankfully, the larger medical system is finally acknowledging the elephant in the exam room. They've got no choice but to do so, because global events in recent years made everyone sit up and take notice. Stress and burnout started happening in record numbers to patients and doctors alike. The healthcare system realized that it was in a pandemic of stress. The silver lining is that we're finally waking up to this reality. The perception of stress management is shifting from something that used to be a luxury, to something that's now considered a necessity for physical and mental health.

If your doctor hasn't asked you about your stress, it's not because they're unaware that stress is a major concern for you right now. Most doctors simply don't have the time, tools, or resources to directly address your stress, especially during a short office visit. They have a long list of pressing medical issues they must monitor in you as their patient: diabetes, heart disease, and the risk of cancer, to name just three common ones. Studies show that for doctors to do their jobs properly, they'd need to work a total of twenty-seven hours a day.[2] Doctors are held to impossible standards and manage a packed agenda with every single office visit. Is it any wonder that a conversation about stress in a doctor's office is sidelined for another day? Ignoring the impact of stress on patient health isn't due to the failings of individual doctors; they're doing the best they possibly can within an overwhelmed system. This is about the systemic failings of a broken healthcare system that prioritizes sick care over health care.

Conventional medical care is finally moving toward acknowledging just how much stress can affect a patient's health. In 2022, a national panel agreed that American adults younger than age sixty-five should be screened for anxiety by their doctor because unhealthy stress is so pervasive, and anxiety is the most common stress-related medical condition.[3] This historic decision could help to transform conventional health care in the near future, but we still have more work to do to build awareness in the medical system about the pervasiveness of stress.

The other big hurdle for doctors, besides their limited time with each patient, is that stress isn't a one-size-fits-all model. Stress shows up differently for each individual, which makes it challenging to identify and treat from the medical perspective. One patient may experience insomnia, headaches, or mood fluctuations, while someone else's stress takes on the form of palpitations, stomach issues, or pain. The list of stress symptoms is vague and vast, which is why we in the medical community call stress a *diagnosis of exclusion*—meaning, before we can label your physical symptom as "stress-related," we first need to exclude all the other possible causes for it, like a medical condition involving your heart, lungs, blood, or brain, among other causes.

If you've had a full medical checkup done and your doctor told you that everything looked okay and your symptoms could be related to stress, you're in good company with those 60 percent to 80 percent of doctors' visits that discover the same thing: it's the stress contributing to the symptoms. Stress has also been found as an aggravating factor in nearly every medical condition, from a benign common cold to a more serious condition like a heart attack. Nearly every medical condition, including anxiety, depression, insomnia, chronic pain, gastrointestinal issues, arthritis, migraines, asthma, allergies, and even diabetes, can be worsened by stress. That's not to say that stress causes these conditions—because that's scientifically inaccurate—but it certainly can make each of them worse.

You might have recognized some of your own stress symptoms in this short list, or maybe your stress shows up in other ways not listed here. After years of studying stress, I can attest to the fact that stress is extremely versatile: it's a multi-hyphenate performer. It can manifest in ways that are both highly unusual and also very common. Sometimes stress can show up as two things at once. Regardless of how stress shows up for you, the first thing I want you to know is that you're not alone. Maybe you've gone a long time trying to ignore your stress symptom or symptoms, but it's now out of hand and you're ready to do something about it.

This was true for Olivia, a married stay-at-home mom of three teen boys, who found her headaches getting worse as her sons were becoming more independent, learning to drive, and staying out later with friends.

As Olivia revealed to me, "I used to have headaches only rarely. Now I'm stressed from raising teenagers, so my headaches happen three or four times every month."

Olivia's doctor had done a complete workup and had determined that the headaches were stress-related, which Olivia didn't feel was very helpful information. "I'm not saying he's wrong, but it doesn't make the headaches any easier to handle," she told me. "I seem to be in a nonstop difficult process of adjusting to my sons and their growing independence. I feel like I have to load them up with precautions to prevent anything bad from happening to them, and then I still worry all the time. They see me as overprotective and are constantly trying to negotiate the rules I set. My oldest is seventeen and the youngest is thirteen. I'll have to pull myself together and get through it, but how will I be with five more years of this headache pain?"

I could see that Olivia was reaching her breaking point.

Like Olivia, most of us have been taught from a young age that tolerating a high level of discomfort is what inner strength is all about. We mistakenly call it resilience. I'm here to tell you, that's not true resilience. What often gets labeled as resilience is the very thing that depletes us in the long run, both physically and mentally. It's what I call the great *resilience myth*.

The Resilience Myth

From a strictly scientific point of view, resilience is your innate biological ability to adapt, recover, and grow in the face of life's challenges. But resilience doesn't function in a vacuum. You need stress for resilience to show itself.

Resilience can be defined as "the ability to cope with shocks and keep functioning in much the same kind of way as before."[14] It is a healthy biological phenomenon. But it's often confused with *toxic resilience*, which is a warped view of this definition and can include unhealthy behaviors like pushing past boundaries, productivity at all costs, and a mind-over-matter mindset. It's the Energizer Bunny mentality, and it can get you into trouble. The foundation of our modern world is built on toxic resilience. As a child in school, you were rewarded for always holding it together. By adulthood, this is the norm whether you're at home, work, parenting, caregiving, or in your community.

I've witnessed this false expectation every day in my clinic. A patient will walk in with a big smile on their face. They seem happy, relaxed, and calm. But then the door closes and they burst into spontaneous tears the moment they have some privacy with me. No matter their age, occupation, or family background, once they feel they can tell the truth about their stress, the floodgates open. It's far too common and a real indicator of just how universal yet isolated we feel in our personal stress struggles. Another aspect of toxic resilience is that we feel shame about needing advice or help, so we resist asking for it until we have no choice. Everyone comes to this realization in their own time.

Miles came to see me at the insistence of his wife because she was concerned with his inability to sleep well. He was sleeping about four hours per night, and for the previous few months he'd been running on fumes most days, with dark circles under his eyes. As a manager of twelve employees in a software engineering division, and with two young children at home, Miles was starting to have other health issues, like high blood pressure.

He perched on the edge of the chair in my office, waiting for the appointment to be over.

"Look, I know my wife is worried," Miles said, trying to make light of it. "I'm going to be fine. I'm under a lot of pressure at work. You know technology. I have to keep up with constant changes. I'm responsible for keeping my division on pace."

"Which has to be difficult if you're going into work without much sleep," I said.

Miles waved the comment away. "Listen doc, I was a champion athlete in college. I would get up to train at four in the morning, every morning. I'm used to pushing through to get results. I'll probably sleep better after things are back on track at work and once my kids are a little older and not as dependent."

"In the meantime, there are some simple techniques that could help you feel better now," I offered.

"I'm sure those are great for your other patients," Miles said, "but I'm okay. My dad never missed a single day of work. I'm built from sturdy stock. I'm only here because my wife asked me to see you. So it was nice to meet you, doctor. Have a great week."

I wished Miles well and watched him walk back out through the waiting room.

Miles was primed with another aspect of toxic resilience. We've learned to tell ourselves that we'll engage in self-care at some future time—when we aren't so busy, when the kids are grown, when we've reached a work goal, when the pressure is off, when we have a vacation week, when there's more money in the bank, when we retire. Regrettably, we give self-care the least attention when we need it the most.

Toxic resilience has been around a long time. In the depths of the Great Depression, the politician Al Smith is credited with saying, "The American people never carry an umbrella. They prepare to walk in eternal sunshine." Eternal sunshine is a lot of pressure to live up to, and it's the perfect slogan for a culture that rewards toxic resilience. This book isn't about learning to walk in eternal sunshine. That's not realistic, feasible, or even sustainable.

Unlike Miles, you may be at a place where you've realized that the levels of stress and burnout in your life are no longer sustainable. You want to see measurable and daily improvements in the way you feel. In the chapters that follow, I give you all the tools you need to create tangible and concrete change so you can overcome your unhealthy stress and reveal your innate and wondrous resilience—the real kind.

The Canary in the Coal Mine

Let's start by redefining your relationship to stress through a short exercise that helps you identify the problem that's disrupting your life the most. It's called the canary in the coal mine.

Coal miners in the nineteenth century took canaries into the mines with them to monitor the amount of deadly carbon monoxide in the air. The miners couldn't tell, on their own, if the air quality was getting into a danger zone, but the canary could. By listening to the canary sing, the miners would know the air was toxic if the bird fell silent. Without paying attention to the canary's song, the workers might have pushed past their limits, risking their health and well-being—even their lives. The canary always alerted the miners before permanent, long-lasting damage had been done to them, before they hit a point of no return.[5]

We human beings are notoriously bad at knowing our limits, and even when we do know them, we often exceed them. We each have a canary within us that signals danger—when we're moving in the wrong direction with our stress. It lets us know when our lifestyle isn't working in our best interest and that we should take action to make change before things move too far in the wrong direction. The canary song that got my attention was my palpitations. They made me sit up, take notice, and make changes in my life and how I lived it. My patients' canaries have alerted them to their stress through insomnia, anxiety, depression, headaches, allergies, heartburn, nausea, dizziness, pain, or recurrent flares of an existing medical condition. Symptoms such as these can tell you it's time to pay attention, slow down, give yourself a little compassion, and make a change.

Like many of my patients, you may have hit your limit and can't ignore your own signs, your canary song. Your symptoms have become a problem for you. But realizing that you need to sit up, take notice, and want to make a change, is what brought you to the techniques in this book. Your canary's song is letting you know it's not too late to get your life back. Within these pages you'll find the directions you need to get out of the dark cave of stress and burnout and finally give yourself that breath of much-needed fresh air.

Let's begin with a short quiz of five questions in which you can get an overview on your own stress level, your own Personalized Stress Score. The questions are very similar to ones that I would ask you during an office visit. But since we aren't together, in person, I want you to have a way to qualify your own starting point to less stress and burnout.

Try your best to answer all five questions as accurately as you

YOUR STRESS SCORE

1. In the past month, how often have you noticed your canary's warning signs?

Never (0) Almost never (1) Sometimes (2) Fairly often (3) Very often (4)

2. In the past month, how often have you felt overloaded or unsettled by your stress?

Never (0) Almost never (1) Sometimes (2) Fairly often (3) Very often (4)

3. In the past month, how often have you felt depleted or low energy because of your stress?

Never (0) Almost never (1) Sometimes (2) Fairly often (3) Very often (4)

4. In the past month, how often have you experienced disrupted sleep because of your stress?

Never (0) Almost never (1) Sometimes (2) Fairly often (3) Very often (4)

5. In the past month, how often have you felt that stress has interfered with your day-to-day life and everyday activities?

Never (0) Almost never (1) Sometimes (2) Fairly often (3) Very often (4)

can. Take your time and think through how each question applies broadly to your life over the past month. Then add up the numbers in parentheses to discover your Personalized Stress Score.

Your Personalized Stress Score can offer you a glimpse into how your stress may be affecting your everyday life. This stress quiz isn't meant to diagnose or treat your stress, but rather, as an educational tool that can give you some insight into how stress manifests for you.[6] Does your stress feel healthy, manageable, and contained—in proportion to the demands of your everyday life? Or does it feel like runaway stress, imbalanced and out of proportion to your everyday life? Your Personalized Stress Score can help you discern the differences in how adaptive stress and maladaptive stress may be showing up for you. The lowest possible score is 0 and the highest you can score is 20. You'll notice that the higher the score, the higher the likelihood of maladaptive stress, and the lower your score, the lower the likelihood of maladaptive stress. Now that you have your initial Personalized Stress Score in hand, how do you feel? Surprised, overwhelmed, confused? Or maybe all of these?

When my patients have answered these questions as a check-in for their stress, they're often disheartened by their high scores. The first thing they say is, "But I'm resilient! I'm not supposed to feel stressed. That doesn't happen to people like me." Does that sound familiar? Yeah, it does to me too. Those were the same words I said to my doctor during my own stress struggle. The truth is, an unhealthy amount of stress can happen to anyone, and the first step to overcoming it is to have a healthy dose of self-compassion as you navigate this new world.

Here's the good news: no matter what your stress score is today, you have the power to change it with small but mighty adjustments. We're going to walk the path to less stress together. With each step, we'll make simple tweaks that work with your biology, rather than against it, to get to your destination of healthy stress.

I've asked my patients similar questions to those within this stress quiz over the years, and they've become helpful guideposts for my patients to gauge their unhealthy stress levels along their stress journey. In the same way you'd monitor your blood pressure regularly, I invite you to retake the stress quiz every four weeks and check in on how your stress score is improving. It's highly motivating to see that score start decreasing because of the changes you make, as it's been for my patients when they've used The 5 Resets in their lives. You'll be amazed just how quickly your brain and body respond to these techniques to rewire your brain for less unhealthy stress and more authentic and long-lasting resilience.

You might be thinking that many of your life's stressors can't be changed, at least not now. I get it. It's not like you can stop paying your bills, ask your boss to change personalities, turn your aging parents into young people again, or snap your fingers and have your toddler potty-trained, your house clean, and add an extra five hours to your day. The purpose of The 5 Resets is to help you navigate your real-life stresses in real time. Retreats, spas, and personal days are great, but measurable progress in overcoming your everyday stress happens when you apply these techniques to your messy, everyday life.

The Tea Kettle of Stress

I'm a tea drinker. In the mornings, I have a strong cup of Irish Breakfast tea with fresh grated ginger, a little brown sugar, and a splash of cold almond milk. I sip my tea and practice my Sticky Feet (a technique you'll learn about in Chapter 6). It's a morning ritual that keeps me grounded in the calm of the moment, helps me plan my day, and primes my brain and body for what's ahead. It's my morning reset.

One day, as I was waiting for the water to boil, I thought about the parallels of the humble tea kettle and my own experiences with unhealthy stress over the years. Even though my nightly wild horse stampede during my medical training was my only experience with acutely debilitating stress, I've been through many experiences over the years that created unhealthy stress for me. Studying for board exams, moving to a new city, and buying my first home were high-pressure times when stress began to gradually accumulate in my body to unhealthy levels. I would feel on edge, be unable to relax and wind down, and occasionally suffer from fitful sleep that left me exhausted the next day. I knew I had very little control over these external events, but because I'd been through my stress episode with the wild horses, I was especially attuned to any signs of unhealthy stress in my body. I now knew that I could control my internal experience of these events, offset my stress, and prevent it from accumulating by using certain scientific principles and techniques.

As I waited to brew my morning tea almost two decades after that first incident with the wild horses, it came to me that our bodies are like tea kettles when it comes to a buildup of unhealthy stress. I realized that my various stressful experiences over the years had taught me effective ways to practice the techniques to release some therapeutic steam. They prevented my unhealthy levels of stress from boiling over.

When you're experiencing unhealthy stress in your life, consider how a tea kettle works on a hot stove. As the water heats, steam builds up inside the kettle. You can lower the heat by turning down the burner, but the reality of our lives is that most of our stresses—such as work, child or elder care, health issues, and school—are external and can't be changed in the moment. Our attempts to change our external environment aren't always in our control or they don't go as planned. We often lose our sense of agency, which can leave us feeling powerless. So we give up on our attempts to control our stress, believing that we must tolerate it or learn to live with it no matter how we feel. But there's another, better way!

If we stop focusing on the external, unchangeable factors and instead put our energy into changing our internal environment, the water inside the tea kettle, change is possible in spite of the heat. We can feel better by releasing the buildup of stress, like opening the lever on the tea kettle's spout to release steam. The 5 Resets will teach you how to release that therapeutic steam.

The Stress Paradox

When I was overwhelmed with my own stress as a medical resident, I took a class that was offered to doctors on staying mindful and present during stressful moments. (You'll learn a technique from this class in Chapter 5.) In an early session of Mindfulness for Healthcare Providers, my teacher, Dr. Michael Baime, told our group, "You know the intensity you're feeling as you're living your life? Every single person feels that same intensity living *their* life. Remember that as you move through the world as a doctor treating patients."

That moment crystallized something deep for me. I've thought about his words often. How can something like stress, which makes a person feel so very alone, also be happening to millions of people simultaneously?

Stress is the most common and unifying experience we have as human beings. We're all living life with the same intensity, but we go through the experience feeling completely alone. *We're completely isolated in our togetherness with stress.* It's one of humankind's greatest paradoxes.

Years later, as a doctor with a busy medical practice, I'd look around my packed waiting room in the hospital and think to myself, "If only my patients could talk to each other, they'd feel less alone because they'd discover that every person here is suffering from the same thing, each in their own way."

According to data from 2015, if you're in a room with thirty people, at least twenty-one of them are likely feeling stressed and burned out *just like you.*[7] That's not to minimize your individual struggle with stress. Each journey is unique and valid. But if we understood exactly how unifying the impact of unhealthy stress has been for so many of us, we'd be able to normalize the experience, which would minimize the shame and isolation we feel about it in the first place.

In clinical medicine, the act of naming a difficult experience and sharing your story with others with the same lived experience is the basis of group therapy. Being a part of a group and sharing similar stories can help you heal and be deeply therapeutic. In scientific terms, it's called the *group effect*. Unfortunately, what I've seen in my everyday experience with patients is the anti–group effect when it comes to stress. Millions of us feel stressed, but no one wants to be identified as someone who is stressed, which shows you just how entrenched the resilience myth is in our culture. I wonder how different things would be if we routinely encouraged group therapy for stress and burnout in the medical setting? Offering free group therapy for everyday stress and burnout would bring people together in a powerful and validating way, helping to unify the many people who struggle alone with their stress. Consider this book as group therapy for your stress.

A Global Snapshot of Stress and Burnout

The rise in stress around the world has accelerated in recent times. Back in 2001, the World Health Organization estimated that one in four people was at risk for developing a stress-related disorder in their lifetime like anxiety, depression, and insomnia.[8] By 2019, the WHO declared burnout an "occupational phenomenon" and designated it as an official clinical syndrome.[9] This was big news at the time, and the new designation helped validate an experience many workers were having and continue to have today. Some might say that stress was the original pandemic. If there's one silver lining from the events of our recent past, it's that stress and burnout are finally getting the recognition they deserve in the world.

It's hard to overstate the impact the past few years have had on our individual and collective stress and burnout. In one survey conducted in February 2022, almost two-thirds of Americans said their lives were forever changed by the COVID-19 pandemic.[10] And another 2022 survey found that mental health has replaced the pandemic as Americans' top health concern.[11] Nearly 70 percent of people feel that the past several years have been the most stressful of their entire professional careers, and nearly that percentage again of people experience at least one feature of burnout.[12] This has led, in part, to an eightfold increase in serious mental distress, including an increase in stress-related disorders like anxiety, depression, and insomnia.[13] Amidst this backdrop, there's been a growing and unmet need for mental health services.[14]

Recent years have also broadened our understanding of what constitutes burnout. What was once considered a purely occupational phenomenon is now infiltrating every sector of life, including parenting and caregiving. In one recent survey, nearly 70 percent of parents reported experiencing burnout.[15] As a parent myself, I can attest to this wholeheartedly, and my hunch is that the real extent of parenting burnout may be far greater.

When envisioning someone with burnout, you're likely to imagine a person with classic characteristics like lack of motivation or feeling disengaged and apathetic. But what modern-day burnout looks like has changed. In one study, 61 percent of people working remotely from home during the pandemic said they found it difficult to disconnect from work even in the presence of burnout.[16] This new face of burnout is what's making it harder to identify it in yourself and others, just like my resilient friend Liz, whom you met at the start of this book.

These bleak statistics aren't meant to get you down but to show you how pervasive stress and burnout are. If you're feeling this way, I hope this helps you see that you aren't alone.

Why Me? Why Now?

Lina had a long history of lupus, a common autoimmune condition. For the previous decade, she had been under the care of an excellent team of capable doctors, while maintaining her full-time job as a court reporter and taking care of her eight-year-old twins as a single mom. Lina made an appointment with me at the recommendation of her mother, who was worried about her daughter's chronic stress. At our first visit, I asked Lina to describe how stress had impacted her body.

Lina was taken aback. "I never thought about how stress works or that it could affect my symptoms," she said. "I just thought my stress and my lupus hung out together without ever talking to each other."

I turned my chair toward hers and said, "I have a question. Do your twins affect each other?"

"Constantly," Lina said. "It's like they're in the same body. If one is in a bad mood, then the other one will be soon. If one starts laughing, the other one does and then they can't stop. They know each other's soft spots, too."

"That's the same with your lupus and your stress," I explained. "Your lupus affects your stress, and your stress affects your lupus."

"I do have more stress when my lupus symptoms are acting up," Lina said.

"Or more stress causes your lupus to get worse," I said. "If you have problems during a court case, what happens with your lupus symptoms that week?"

"Oh, every day has a challenge or two. But if it's a long and complicated case, I make it through my nine-to-five job and then my finger joints swell and turn red over the weekend. And I'm exhausted!"

"It sounds like you hold up during short-term challenges, but when it becomes chronic stress day after day, your body reacts," I said.

"I've had that happen many times," Lina admitted, wide-eyed with the realization of how her stress and lupus symptoms reacted to each other. "And at home, too, like when both the twins came down with strep throat at the same time and couldn't go to school or daycare."

"So you were stuck without help?" I asked.

"Yes. I was so fatigued, in pain, and anxious about calling out of work," she nodded. "I felt like I couldn't handle it, like I was both a bad employee and a bad mom."

"You're not alone in your feelings," I consoled her. "So many people feel this way and suffer in silence, thinking that they're being weak."

Lina shook her head slowly and looked down at her lap. I could see how weary she was in her struggle with stress.

People like Lina, and most likely you as well, are the reason why I wanted to develop a clinical practice focused solely on stress management, especially since 97 percent of people have never had stress management addressed at doctor visits.[17] Lina had spent most of her adult life as a stressed patient within the conventional medical system, yet none of her doctors had explained to her how stress worked in her brain and body.

"Did you want to say something else?" I asked her.

"Yes, but it feels selfish to say because I know horrible things happen to people all the time and my life isn't that bad compared to many other people," Lina said. She turned her face toward the wall. It was obvious that it was difficult for her to say what she next told me.

"Dr. Nerurkar, I try to be a good person, pay my bills, take care of my children, and be there for my mom if she needs help. I guess I feel angry, you know? I already have an autoimmune disease. If that makes my stress worse, and stress makes my symptoms worse, it feels hopeless. I want to know: Why me? Why now? What did I do wrong?"

"Lina, you didn't do anything wrong. Even when we're doing our best to handle life, our brains have a response to stress that is as old as time," I explained.

"Are you telling me that I was born with a response to stress?" she asked.

"That's right," I said. "And it answers the 'why me, why now?' question."

At that point, I gave Lina a quick crash course on how the brain responds to stress, and it opened up a whole new understanding for her. This quick explanation of how the human brain responds to stress has benefited many of my patients, like Lina, and I hope it gives you a deeper understanding of what's happening inside your brain, too.

But before we head into that discussion, I'd like you to begin by allowing some compassion for yourself now that you know stress and burnout are no longer the exception for the majority of people. Even if you were taken aback or disappointed by your Personalized Stress Score, remember that most of us (including me) have been socially conditioned to accept the resilience myth in our lives. We believe we're supposed to be able to push through and handle everything without questioning the myth. Now that you've tuned in to your canary singing and it's become loud and clear, you can't put off caring for yourself in this therapeutic way any longer.

Stress and burnout aren't the exception anymore, they're the rule. The good news is that both stress and burnout are fully reversible.

But before you can get to work on reversing your stress and burnout, it's helpful to understand how your brain responds to chronic stress. You now have more insight into how stress manifests for you outwardly in your daily life, so let's take a look at your biology of stress from the inside out as a way to clearly understand what stress is doing internally to your brain and body. When you know why and how stress and burnout hijacked your brain, you'll find it easier to use the techniques of The 5 Resets to rewire your brain and body for less stress and more resilience.

2

What Your Brain Thinks About Stress

To have the best overview of The 5 Resets, it's helpful for you to have a baseline understanding of what happens to your brain and body during challenging, stressful moments. Your doctor may have never explained the science of stress, but knowing a little more about how unhealthy stress can take aim at your brain and body will help you better understand why it's important to reset and release its grip on you.

Under usual circumstances, when you're not particularly stressed, your brain is led by the *prefrontal cortex*. If you put your palm on your forehead, it's the area of the brain right behind your palm. Your prefrontal cortex helps you manage your day-to-day life decisions. It can plan your kid's birthday party, organize your desktop files, think through how to hang curtains, or in which order to give two presentations at the fall conference. The prefrontal cortex can look at your options and choose renting a van instead of a sedan, whether you should wear business casual or jeans to an event, or even help you make a decision about which jar of pasta sauce to buy at the grocery store. These brain tasks of planning, organizing, and decision-making are known as *general executive functions*. In real life, a lot of what the prefrontal cortex does could be considered "adulting." When you're feeling calm without much stress, you're pretty good at adulting, but under the influence of stress, things can go awry.

Under stress, your brain is led by the *amygdala*, a bean-size structure located deep in the brain. The amygdala is also known as the reptilian brain or lizard brain, because although humans have evolved, this part of the brain has not. The amygdala is cave dweller mode and has been with us since the beginning of time for a very good reason. It's focused on survival and self-preservation, and it's in charge of your fear response. When it senses a threat, the amygdala activates your stress response, called *fight or flight*. It recruits other brain areas like the hypothalamus and pituitary gland to make the hormone cortisol, which activates your adrenal glands to make adrenaline—which helps you either fight a threat or flee from it. These three entities—the hypothalamus, pituitary gland, and adrenal glands—form what we call the *HPA axis*, which is the main highway for stress in your body.

When you're driven by the amygdala on the HPA highway, fear and stress are the dominant mental states. Your heart beats faster, you breathe more quickly, and you become hypervigilant. This fight or flight response has served the human species exceedingly well when cave dwellers were escaping the deadly jaws of predators. But now, the only predators you face are the ones that never seem to let up on the attack: relationship conflicts, job expectations, bills, family pressures, and deadlines of all kinds—so your amygdala stays activated in the background. Your amygdala is your emotional brain, not your logical brain, so even though you may logically understand that a work deadline isn't exactly a life-threatening circumstance, your amygdala can't discern the difference.

If during a moment of heightened panic with a deadline you've felt doom and gloom and said to yourself, “My boss is going to kill me if I don’t finish this,” that’s your amygdala talking.

The modern brain doesn’t get a chance to reset back to normal, baseline levels because of the high levels of chronic stress in your life, like constant deadlines and financial pressures. Stress is what keeps your amygdala active, day in and day out.

Your brain and body were expertly designed to handle acute stress really well, but chronic stress creates an overuse problem for the amygdala and the stress response. You can tolerate cave dweller mode for a short time because your brain and body were designed for survival and self-preservation. But if it goes on for many months or years at a time, burnout can set in. This cognitive glitch is the key to understanding why your stress and burnout have been stuck at unprecedented levels.

A corporation that invited me to speak to their 450 employees about stress sent a young junior associate, David, to pick me up at the airport. As we got to talking while sitting in traffic, David told me about his pandemic experience, working at home for fifteen months, and how his life had been going since his employer had requested everyone return to the office.

“I was stuck in my studio apartment, trying to work on a tiny table in the corner,” David said. “It was okay at first, because they said it would be only two weeks, maybe three. No big deal, right? Then the pandemic ramped up in full and they told us they didn’t know when or if the offices would reopen. I felt totally trapped and isolated.”

“Lots of people are right there with you,” I told David. “We all thought it would be a tiny blip in our lives, a short sprint of laying low and quarantining. Then, reality set in and we were all like ‘Now what?’”

Perhaps you can relate to these feelings. When most of us thought the COVID crisis would be a short-term inconvenience, our brains were primed and ready to handle a limited burst of stress. We all hunkered down and waited for the acute threat to pass. But the threat persisted, with no clear end in sight. The sprint turned into a marathon with no finish line. This was a different beast to our brains, which were no longer in acute threat mode, but rather in chronic threat mode.

We were told to hang in there. For three years, headlines promised us the Roaring Twenties after the pandemic was over. A time of reckless abandon. As I read the articles, I remember thinking, "This is false advertising because that's not how human brains work when it comes to stress."

"It's weird," David said. "I actually feel worse now than when I didn't know if I was going to get sick, or what would happen to my job, or when I'd ever get to fly home to see my family, or even keep up with paying my rent."

I asked David, "In what way do you feel worse?"

"I'm really down. I never was before. And even simple things like responding to work emails or trying to get to the Laundromat and back makes me feel overwhelmed. I mean, you're a doctor. Does it sound like I'm losing it?"

"If you're losing it, then so are millions of people around the world," I answered.

The pandemic marathon led to mental health consequences because the human brain is not meant to sustain large amounts of stress for long periods of time without a reset. "Don't blame yourself. It's not you, it's your biology of stress," I explained to David. "What you're experiencing is a normal, healthy, and expected biological response to chronic stress."

"It's good to hear I'm not just a featherweight. Still, I gotta ask, why now? Now that everything has returned to normal, you'd think

I'd be all good," David said. "But I'm not. I can't seem to man up and get out of this funk."

If the way David feels is close to what you're going through, here's the reason: you're experiencing a *delayed stress response*. During acute crises, your brain rises up to meet the challenge because, as humans, we're hardwired for survival and self-preservation. We always find a way to address our immediate needs. You will rarely find someone in the midst of calamity who is emotionally falling apart for the entirety of the calamity. Of course, it can happen, but it's rare.

Your brain is built like a dam that recognizes acute crisis and holds it all together so that you can do what is needed in the moment. Then once the acute threat has passed and you feel psychologically safe, the dam breaks, you let your guard down, and your true emotions come to the surface. It's a deluge.

Maybe you were perfectly okay during the acute crisis. Perhaps you were even complimented for your ability to hold it together at all costs. But now, you're more irritable, depleted, keyed up, depressed, unfocused, anxious, or all of the above, depending on the day or time. You feel very different from your usual self. It's not a personal choice or a shortcoming; it's your biology. It's how the human brain is designed. I've seen this same delayed stress response play out hundreds of times with so many of my patients. It's why I had the stampede of horses at night after a stressed workday.

"I don't get it," my patient Raquel admitted to me, leaning her head into her hand. "Why am I feeling so upset *now*?" Earlier in the year she had come to see me to help her manage the stress of a new cancer diagnosis. At that time, she was incredibly calm and stoic, and didn't shed a tear. She had a plan in place for surgery, radiation, and chemotherapy. Her oncology team recently had claimed her treatment "a success" and given her a clean bill of health. She was happily discharged from their care and told to follow up for routine care in three months. Then, seven days later she came to see me in my office. She was distraught, anxious, and weeping uncontrollably and very confused by her emotions.

"I just got the good news that I'm cancer-free," she told me with an exasperated sob. "I should be out partying, but I'm a mess. I can't sleep. I've never been so anxious. I have so much doom and gloom. This should be the happiest time of my life! It makes no sense at all."

"Actually, Raquel, this is what happens, and it makes perfect sense," I said, handing her the box of tissues. "During your cancer treatment, your defenses were up. Your psyche was under an acute threat, so you shored up your inner reserves and all of your vigor to get through radiation and chemotherapy for many weeks."

Raquel nodded in relief as I explained to her that once her treatment course was complete and her oncologist gave her the good news, she felt psychologically safe to allow for her true stress response to show itself. Suppressing her emotions during treatment wasn't a conscious or intentional choice on her part; it's just how the human brain is wired to respond to acute threats.

"Look how strong you really are," I told her. "Your psyche overcame the stress of facing cancer and won."

A delayed stress response like Raquel's is a normal and expected part of the healing journey after an acutely stressful event like cancer. But it doesn't have to take a health scare to activate this delayed response. Acute stress or trauma in any aspect of life can bring this about.

I studied the delayed stress response when I worked in refugee health with a WHO Collaborating Center in Geneva, Switzerland. Most of us can't imagine having to flee our homelands, leaving behind everything except whatever we can carry in our arms. Refugees, like those in recent conflicts, appear incredibly resilient as they make their way to a completely unknown future or have to live in tents in refugee camps. It's when they are at long last in a safe place, either a new country or back in their homelands, that many of their true mental health issues surface.[1]

Even without the extremes of a cancer diagnosis or a refugee experience, a delayed stress response can happen to anyone, especially since we've all endured difficult experiences together over the past several years, when our collective mental health took a hit beginning in early 2020. We were mentally prepared for a pandemic sprint, but instead we got a pandemic marathon with an ever-extended finish line. We were unprepared for the cognitive shift, a major change in our thinking, once we understood it wouldn't be over after a couple weeks of quarantine, as originally expected. In doctor-speak, we went from an acute condition to a chronic one. Unfortunately, the result was that our brains had to withstand unusually high levels of stress for an extended period of time.

Now that you know about the delayed stress response, you can see how the high stress, pressure-cooker situation of our collective recent past can be the cause of the rampant burnout and mental health challenges of the present and most likely into the near future.

If there's a ray of light to this dark cloud of traumatic events, it's that we went through the experience together. The fact that so many of us are experiencing the delayed stress response is what makes this moment ripe with the promise of healing and possibility. We now have a huge opportunity to normalize and validate our shared experience and, most important, to reset our stress to a healthy level and overcome our burnout. You now have the perfect opportunity, through The 5 Resets, to make huge positive strides in your stress, resilience, and mental health.

Stress is a whole-body phenomenon. We get waves of negative emotion, the familiar feelings of reaching a boiling point and experiencing doom and gloom. Whatever your sensory experience of stress might be, the origin of stress starts in the same place—the brain. Specifically, stress starts in an area called the *hippocampus* in the brain's limbic system, according to scientists at Yale University.[2] The limbic system is your emotional center, and the hippocampus is responsible for learning and memory. So if stress is born in the same place as learning and memories are made, stress can be considered a learned response. And as with any learned response, *it can be unlearned* and retrained in a better way. That's the first premise of why your brain can be rewired for less stress.

The second scientific principle behind rewiring your brain for less stress is based on one of the greatest discoveries in brain science: *neuroplasticity*. Before your eyes glaze over with this doctor-speak, it's just a fancy word for your brain's ability to change.

It turns out that your brain is a muscle that grows and changes on the basis of the ever-changing conditions of your life. This applies to different parts of the brain, the connections between areas of the brain, and even among individual brain cells. If your biceps can get stronger by doing bicep curls, you can also train the muscle of the brain. It's like pumping iron, but in this case pumping neurons. Your neurons, or nerve cells, make connections with each other to carry and transmit updated and new information between areas of the brain and throughout your body's entire nervous system. They are good at finding the quickest route between two points, but it takes a number of trips to really establish a solid new connection. The brain is always establishing new routes and, the good news is, for the most part you can choose to strengthen the helpful ones through repetition. The more you engage in a new habit, the stronger that brain pathway becomes. Neuroplasticity is the phenomenon of your brain being able to change on the basis of what it experiences and is the foundation for this book.

Before the discovery of neuroplasticity, the scientific community thought that the brain you were born with would be the same brain you'd be stuck with for life. Yup, a real grab bag. But through new brain imaging techniques like functional magnetic resonance imaging (fMRI) and electroencephalography (EEG) we've learned that the brain's structure, cells, and connections grow or shrink according to your behaviors.[3] Neuroplasticity is what gives you the ability to rewire your brain.

As you gradually begin to train your brain for less stress and more resilience, it's important to keep in mind what I call the *Resilience Rule of 2.* Your brain is a muscle, just like your biceps. You wouldn't dream of bench pressing one hundred pounds of iron without working up to it. Well, your brain also needs to gradually work itself up to being reshaped. You need to give yourself a little practice to pump your neurons too.

It's tempting to go fast, but when you use the Resilience Rule of 2 to make slow and gradual changes to your brain—only two at a time—the changes become easier to incorporate into your everyday life and don't feel as difficult. And those changes are more likely to stick around for the long term and become a part of who you are, rather than something you do every once in a while.

The Resilience Rule of 2

My patient Adam was hell-bent on fixing his stress problem when he came to see me in early March. From the outsider's perspective, he looked like a man in control. His business was growing year to year, and he had a busy family life raising two teenage daughters with his wife. Adam was a self-described achiever, "striving for excellence" in anything he set his mind to. And he had recently set his sights on fixing his stress once and for all.

"Here's the deal. I was feeling super burned out last year," Adam declared. "I knew I had to make changes, so my New Year's resolution was to go full court press on my stress."

Adam showed me a three-ring binder that was at capacity with a hundred pages of stress interventions he'd already tried. "I'm hacking my way to less stress," he said.

Determined to make a radical change, Adam had completely overhauled his lifestyle starting on January 1. He had a checklist for his sleep, food, exercise, and energy levels. If it was trackable, he was logging it. He had kept this up, on his own, for about two months, but his enthusiasm was waning. His determination had turned into another source of stress.

As he closed his binder, he seemed defeated. "I'm here because I can't do it anymore," he told me. "I was doing everything all at once. I didn't know what was working and what wasn't. It's frustrating."

"This is how our biology reacts during huge lifestyle overhauls," I said. "We've been misled to believe that a person can and should make a lot of radical changes quickly. But what happens is our biology rebels against trying to change too much too fast."

"Probably the reason most New Year's resolutions don't last," Adam said.

"Exactly," I concurred. "We set these all-or-nothing resolutions and end up feeling worse about ourselves when we can't keep it up."

"I noticed that on January 2, my gym was packed at seven thirty in the morning," Adam said. "Yesterday, there were only about eight of us using the machines. I used to go every day. Now, I'm really pissed at myself because I make it there only twice a week."

I assured him that his declining enthusiasm and sense of overwhelm were normal and expected. There was nothing wrong with him; in fact, there was everything right with him. His biology was working exactly as it should during a huge lifestyle overhaul. "It's the Resilience Rule of 2," I explained. "It's why we can't make too many changes at once if we want those changes to stick—no matter how enthusiastic and ready we are for them!"

When it comes to how your brain responds to change, even positive change registers as stress to your brain. You may have the best of intentions to improve yourself, like Adam did, but you can make only two new changes at a time if you want those changes to last and be sustainable. Anything more than two at once and your system has a higher risk of overload. It wasn't Adam's fault that he couldn't keep up with his plan. It wasn't a lack of discipline or motivation. It was his biology.

The fact that your brain registers even positive life changes as stress was discovered by two researchers in the 1960s. Drs. Thomas Holmes and Richard Rahe were two psychiatrists who wanted to understand how life changes affected stress and health. They studied five thousand patients and picked forty-three of the most common life events to determine whether the event led to stress.[4] The events ran the gamut, from graduating school to getting a new job, buying a home, achieving an outstanding personal goal, getting married, having a child, getting divorced, retiring, and experiencing the death of a loved one. Each life event, both challenging ones and joyful ones, had a particular score. The more life events a person accrued, the higher their stress score and the greater the likelihood of their developing an illness.

This landmark study solidified our understanding of life stress and the brain. It showed us that even "positive life changes still require some effort to adapt and regain stability" and therefore could have negative stress consequences.[5] My approach to patients is built on this understanding. Even changes for the better, the good kind of change, can be perceived as stress by the brain and body.

I was taught early in my medical training that if I wanted my patients to make positive changes to their lives, such as having better sleep habits, improving their diet, or quitting smoking, I could recommend only two new changes at a time if I wanted those changes to be sustainable in a patient's life. Otherwise, there was a greater chance that the changes wouldn't stick. The basis for this approach comes from the early work of Holmes and Rahe almost sixty years ago, and doctors have applied these findings ever since to help their patients make lasting, positive lifestyle changes. Through my research on stress, I realized that it was significant for patients to have a clear understanding of the concept so they could apply it to their lives. I began to call it the Resilience Rule of 2.

Adam may have wanted to hack stress by using the everything-but-the-kitchen-sink philosophy, but I advised him to try the Resilience Rule of 2 instead. We focused on two key areas in his life that needed attention: sleep and exercise. I gave him my resets for both (which you'll learn in Chapters 4 and 5), and he was able to follow both because his mental bandwidth wasn't tied up with any other changes.

So Adam and I started out with two simple techniques. When he came to see me for his follow-up a few months later, we added two more changes.

Since the changes were introduced gradually, two at a time, his brain had time to adapt to the stress, even if it was the good kind. And that made all the difference.

Your Lifestyle Snapshot

When I saw Adam in my office, I was able to ask him a series of questions to gather all the information I needed to craft his personalized stress-management prescription. Through a long conversation, Adam answered the questions on my lifestyle inventory, and together we created his plan of care. My clinical decision-making includes many such conversations with my patients, along with other pertinent data, such as their medical conditions, symptoms, and preferences, so that I can tailor a stress-management prescription targeted to their individual needs.

Even though I can't speak one-on-one with you, you can think of this book as our conversation. I want to simulate for you the experience that my patients have with me during an appointment.

To do this, take a few minutes to take a Lifestyle Snapshot. Ask yourself the same questions I would ask you if you came to see me in the clinic—questions about your sleep, media use, sense of community, exercise, and diet. When you see your written responses, you can get a clearer picture of where you are at this moment—which aspects of your life you are excelling at, and which areas need a little improvement. Once you have your Lifestyle Snapshot, then you can go through The 5 Resets and their corresponding strategies and fold them into your life.

YOUR LIFESTYLE SNAPSHOT

Your Sleep

Bedtime

- What time do you get into bed? ________
- What time do you fall asleep? ________
- What activities do you do two hours before bedtime? ________
- Do you have difficulty falling asleep? ________
- Do you have difficulty staying asleep? ________

Awakening

- What time do you wake up? ________
- What time do you physically get out of bed? ________
- Do you wake up feeling rested? ________

Sleep Quality

- Do you have fragmented sleep? ________
- If yes, approximately how many nights per week? ________

Your Media Use

- How many hours per day total do you spend in front of a screen (this includes your phone, computer, television, and other electronic devices with screens)? ________
- How often do you check your phone for emails, social media, or messages (for instance, about every half hour, every hour, or every few hours)? ________
- Do you check your phone for emails, social media or messages first thing in the morning before getting out of bed? ________
- Do you wake up at night to check your phone for emails, social media, or messages? ________

Your Sense of Community

Home Environment

- Do you live alone or with others? ________
- If you live with others, how would you characterize your relationships with them? ________

Social Network

- Do you feel like you have family members or friends whom you can depend on? ________
- Do you feel a sense of community? ________
- If you had an emergency at four o'clock in the morning, are there at least two people you could call for help? ________

Your Movement Inventory

- How many times per week do you exercise, on average? ________
- What kind of exercise do you do? ________
- How long is each exercise session? ________

Your Daily Diet

- Do you minimize eating processed foods? ________
- Do you crave processed foods and sweets (like cookies, potato chips, and cake) on a regular/daily basis? ________
- Do you engage in emotional eating, that is, eating when you're bored, stressed, or tired? ________
- Does your diet include vegetables, fruits, lean proteins, and whole grains? ________
- Are you on any special diets? ________

You've now taken an important step in demystifying your stress by bringing your regular routines and habits into sharper focus with a Lifestyle Snapshot. Because unhealthy stress is incrementally compounded or reduced through such habits, it's helpful to have this snapshot of what you do most days. When it comes to the difference between healthy and unhealthy stress, as author and podcaster Gretchen Rubin says, "What you do every day matters more than what you do once in a while."[6]

Unhealthy stress is caused by many overlapping factors—not just one thing—but when you hear your canary sing and you feel its effects, your habits can become a tangled mess. When your stressed brain is in survival mode being led by your amygdala, it's hard to discern whether your regular habits are helping you or hurting you. You're left in a jumble of heightened emotions, trying to make it through each day.

Taking a Lifestyle Snapshot and looking at it carefully starts to shift your brain out of survival mode and into thriving mode, which is led by the prefrontal cortex. Your Lifestyle Snapshot is an overview of where you currently are, and the fifteen techniques within The 5 Resets are the way to where you want to be. You can use those techniques to rewire your brain and body for less stress and more resilience.

As tempting as it may be to bring all the techniques into your life immediately, similar to what Adam was trying to do, try to work with your biology by using the Resilience Rule of 2. Begin with two techniques at a time, and once you're feeling good about them, add two more. Otherwise, your road to less stress will feel, well, too stressful. Change is tricky for the brain and body, so go slow and try to keep a healthy dose of patience as you proceed. Your experience reading this book, for instance, should feel calm, healing, and therapeutic—what has long been called *bibliotherapy*—and not add to your stress!

Patience is needed because it takes a little longer than eight weeks to create a new habit. (You'll learn more about the science of habits in Chapter 5.) A visual record of your progress can help, so as you're starting out, keep a checklist of your progress. You can be as high-tech or low-tech as you wish with your checklist. Some of my patients use paper and pen, others use a calendar, and others use an app. Whatever your mode to record your reset, use it daily to help strengthen the brain pathways of habit formation. After your initial enthusiasm slows down, you may need a nudge to keep going. Having a visual cue, like a checkmark that you can complete every day, can be a gratifying push in the right direction.

The magic of The 5 Resets is that they are practical, actionable strategies firmly rooted in science: by working with your biology rather than against it, you can optimize your ability to make healthy, lasting changes to your stress, burnout, and mental health. You'll soon feel the satisfaction of success.

3

The First Reset: Get Clear on What Matters Most

How great would it be if the Google Maps or Waze apps on our phones could give us real-time directions for how to change our unhealthy stress? We could relax and know that we would arrive at a better place one or two suggestions at a time.

These navigation apps on our phones work because we know where we are starting and where we want to go. Once we tell the app our destination, the technology gives us step-by-step instructions on the easiest way to get there. Even though I don't have a voice-activated solution for your stress and burnout, the First Reset is all about your getting clear on your destination—what matters most, your personal priority—and getting you into the right mindset to easily arrive at that destination.

Perhaps you're thinking "I don't know where to begin." That's not uncommon. Stress and burnout have jumbled your navigation tools and left you adrift. So the very first step is to shift your brain circuitry from survival mode into a healthier mental state of psychological safety and self-trust. Together, we'll cover three techniques—Uncovering Your MOST Goal, Creating Your Backwards Plan, and Finding Your Buried Treasure—to help you crystallize your goals for less stress. Let's discover what matters most to you by bringing it into sharper focus with this First Reset.

Stepping into Your Growth Mindset

I want you to know that as much as stress is a part of your biology, so is resilience. No exception. No matter how far from resilient you may feel right now, it's still an innate part of who you are. It may be dormant and buried deep inside you today, but through the techniques in this book you'll uncover your resilience over the next few months. I've witnessed it with countless patients in my clinic, and I believe in your success story, too. Stick with me!

The most empowering aspect of this relationship between stress and resilience is that if your brain can be taught how to experience less stress, it can also be taught how to build more resilience. Though resilience is an innate quality within you, only time, patience, and practice can strengthen it. You may be a bit anxious and uncoordinated at first, like when you first learned to swim; but surprisingly, you need the presence of healthy stress for your resilience to show itself.

Healthy stress is the swim instructor who pushes you to make it to the edge of the pool on your own, and resilience is what keeps your head above the water, even if your arms are flailing around the first time. With time and patience, you're going to be gliding through the water with strong, confident strokes even when healthy stress challenges you.

Since our brains have the biological ability to physically change, adapt, and grow to serve us better, it also means that you as a person have that same ability. Embracing the idea that change can help you become wiser, stronger, and more adaptable is the essence of the *growth mindset*. You may have heard of the growth mindset in corporate or business settings, but this mindset is highly applicable to your mental health too. The growth mindset is your brain's workaround from unhealthy stress to healthy stress, and it uses your innate resilience to stay in motion.

Moving Through the Three Zones of Fear, Learning, and Growth

When Jeanette came to see me, she was convinced that her brain couldn't change. "I think my brain is permanently broken," she said, thumping her cane on the floor in frustration.

Jeanette, a fifty-eight-year-old apartment building manager, had suffered a recent stroke, affecting her ability to walk well. After a short hospitalization, she had continued going to physical therapy every week, but the whole ordeal had understandably caused a lot of stress.

"I've tried to reduce my stress in all kinds of ways, but nothing's fixing it," she told me.

I asked Jeanette why she went to weekly physical therapy appointments. "Because they're teaching me to walk again," she said. "Two months ago, I could barely walk down a hallway. Now, I can walk around the block. I may not need this cane much longer."

"That's incredible progress in two months!" I said. "If you can learn to walk again, then your brain isn't broken."

Jeanette started to smile. "Well, my partner will be happy to hear that. We're hoping to go on a cruise with some friends this spring."

"I think that's a wonderful goal, Jeanette. Your brain has the capacity to do amazing things. We're going to start physical therapy for your brain together!"

We laughed at the thought of it, but it was the truth. The work we were about to embark on was like physical therapy for Jeanette's stressed brain. In the same way the muscles in her legs were learning to balance and walk again, her brain was a muscle that would soon learn to have healthy stress.

I could see in Jeanette's eyes that she was feeling more hopeful and was starting to believe in her brain's ability to change. We began our work right then and there.

Jeanette was already living in the Growth Zone. She just didn't know it yet.

You may have heard of the Comfort Zone. But there are three other zones that we move through when we're faced with an acute stress or unexpected circumstances that push us out of our Comfort Zone: the Fear Zone, the Learning Zone, and the Growth Zone.[1]

Jeanette had entered the Fear Zone because of her unexpected stroke. At first, she spiraled into a panic. She was initially unable to walk on her own, and this naturally overwhelmed her. She couldn't imagine how she'd ever be able to do daily, routine things again. Thoughts of being permanently disabled led her amygdala to remain in constant survival mode. In the Fear Zone, Jeanette's ability to reorient herself toward a better future was limited.

Over the next two months, with the support of her physician team and physical therapists, Jeanette began to stand on her own and take steps with a walker. Her confidence increased gradually, and soon she was walking down the hallway with her cane and then around the block. She felt less afraid and more in control. Jeanette was heading into her Learning Zone.

Jeanette had already begun her efforts toward recovery, but in the Learning Zone her amygdala settled down and her brain slowly accepted the fact that she didn't have to live in fight-or-flight mode any longer. Her brain's neuroplasticity had already kicked in. She was learning how to manage the limitations created by her unexpected situation. In the Learning Zone, Jeanette was able to shift her focus and attention away from survival mode and into improving her circumstances day by day.

At her first visit with me, Jeanette was at the beginning of her Growth Zone. She had made significant progress with her physical challenges and wanted to make the same progress in her stress. She was now ready to bring The 5 Resets into her life. In the Growth Zone, Jeanette had started to create sense and derive meaning from her difficult situation. She reflected on her recent difficulties and how she had worked to overcome them. She was open to the new challenge of learning how to reset her stress because, having recently overcome a challenge, her self-efficacy had gone up. She had more confidence in her skills and ability to reset her stress.

The three zones are a gradual, progressive journey we all take during setbacks. First, there's the unexpected change that causes acute stress (Fear Zone). Our brains then move past survival mode and we gradually learn ways to adapt to this change (Learning Zone). Finally, we gain a new perspective from the experience (Growth Zone). One way or another, we learn something new from what we've been through. It doesn't have to be an acute physical stress, such as Jeanette's stroke. It can be a wide scope of unexpected changes: a job loss, having to move, the end of a relationship, the death of a loved one, a natural disaster, a dramatic change in finances, or discovering that a long-held belief isn't true. What causes acute stress for one person can be very different from what causes it for someone else.

Like Jeanette, you've also been using the Growth Zone mindset without knowing it. In the wake of the pandemic, one universal experience that you very likely shared with others was being thrown into an unexpected change that created acute stress. In March 2020, you probably started your pandemic quarantine in a state of fear or panic, along with everyone else. Because it was a new unknown and felt like an immediate danger, your brain's self-preservation mechanism automatically went into overdrive. Your primal fear for safety was stoked, especially since there were no quick solutions to defeating this life-threatening virus. Was it going to get much worse? No one knew. Many of us lived in this scary mindset and Fear Zone for most of 2020. It's what compelled some people to hoard toilet paper and hand sanitizer.

By 2021 and into 2022, your brain had slowly adapted to the changes. You learned to put boundaries around your fear, so it no longer consumed your waking hours. You likely were still frightened of the many unknowns—I know I was, even though I'm trained in public health. But you developed skills to contain your fears. You became aware of ways you could protect your health, which you hopefully used. Through your lived experience, you gradually, and unknowingly, moved out of the Fear Zone and into a new Learning Zone. Your path from fear to learning may have been messy and fraught with challenges, but you did it.

By 2023 and 2024, we had entered the postpandemic Growth Zone. Your brain and body may not have fully processed what you had gone through or the ways it changed your life. Even after the threat and restrictions passed, the aftereffects brought on high levels of stress and burnout for many of us. We had lived through the perfect storm with one stress after another without respite, including other recent events that left us feeling vulnerable.

As proficient as the brain and body are at managing stress, they still need time to recover and recalibrate. Without that time, one source of stress compounds another, leading to more stress. Because of this cycle, you may be feeling depleted and wary of your next step. I'm here to lock arms with you and walk forward through the Growth Zone, where you can get a wide-angle view of where you've been, process what you've experienced, and navigate your brighter future. It's closer than you think.

The Science of Action

When you're feeling stressed and burned out, it's easy to fall into the trap of negative self-talk. You may feel blame and shame. You may ask yourself, "What's the matter with me?" You've learned about the paradox of stress—that is, stress being such an isolating experience despite the fact that we all experience it. But as we've seen, when it comes to the very human experience of stress, there's nothing wrong with you and everything right with you. As one of my favorite meditation teachers, Jon Kabat-Zinn, often says, "As long as you are breathing, there is more right with you than wrong with you."[2]

I help people every day to turn their negative self-talk into something that's more compassionate and helpful. In fact, it's something I practice in my own life when I feel offtrack.

One day, early in my stress struggle, when I was mired in negative self-talk, I walked into a used bookstore and saw a tattered copy of the 1971 book by psychologist Mildred Newman and her husband Bernard Berkowitz, *How to Be Your Own Best Friend*. The title made me laugh, and for that reason alone I bought it. I loved that little book. Published before I was born, it felt like my wise grandparents' insights were being imparted to me whenever I read it, which I did often. I was raised by my grandparents in Mumbai during my early years and that old-time wisdom felt comforting during a time of confusion and chaos in my life. But wow, did I get a lot of good-natured flack and jostling from my family and friends for carrying around that little book like a security blanket. To this day, my brother loves reminding me to be my own best friend. The thing is, the book did its job. I don't need the reminder anymore.

When you ruminate on your stress and think "What's the matter with me?," you may be getting only negative and defeating answers to the question. You are most likely far more critical of yourself than anyone else would be of you or you would be of anyone else.

To get out of this habit of negative self-talk, ask yourself the question that will help you silence your negative self-talk and get you into the Growth Zone: instead of asking "What's the matter *with* me?" ask, "What matters most *to* me?" That's what Dr. Edward Phillips, founder of the Institute of Lifestyle Medicine and Whole Health Medical Director at VA Boston Healthcare System, encourages his patients to ask themselves. He emphasizes that we can only make changes that align with what matters most to us.

When Wes came to see me, he was caught up in his negative self-talk and unable to make a change. He worked two jobs and single-parented his three children with the help of his mother and father. He had many obligations on his time and felt like he wasn't making headway in any area of his life, mostly only keeping pace. He felt his stress was catching up to him and would soon affect his long-term health.

Wes's doctors were concerned about his increasing weight because of his history of high cholesterol and high blood pressure. As we talked in my office, Wes came to the conclusion that to care for his children, he had to focus on his health.

"Right now, losing weight is what matters most to me," Wes told me. "I want to stay healthy, but I've been heading in the wrong direction and putting on the pounds."

"I eat fast food twice a day," he admitted, "even though I promised myself I was going to stop. I'll be slamming myself for having no self-control and then I'll go all the way in, eating chips and candy from the vending machines at work."

"I get it," I said to Wes. "You feel stuck in a pattern."

"Truth," Wes said. "And I can't seem to get out of my own way."

Wes worked a desk job during normal business hours and was also a security guard in the evenings. His mother and father picked up his kids from school, helped them with their homework and dinner, and then put them to bed. Wes spoke to his children on the phone every night from the parking lot of a burger chain, which was the closest restaurant between his two jobs and where he'd stop for a quick dinner.

Wes was doing the best he could.

"I know a burger and fries aren't the healthiest things to eat for dinner every night," he told me, "but it's easy and cheap and doesn't interfere with speaking to my kids."

Before our conversation that day, his doctors had encouraged Wes to lose weight, but they didn't have the time to fully delve into understanding the mechanics of his life. Wes didn't suffer from a gap in knowledge or information. He had all the knowledge and information he needed about why weight loss had to be his top health priority. In fact, he had been bombarded by it during his doctors' visits and in his own online searches. But many of the strategies he read about online about how to lose weight seemed out of touch with and not directly applicable to his lifestyle. He couldn't spend hours at the gym, eat salads every day, or have home-cooked dinners instead of eating out.

Because Wes was stressed and feeling the intense burdens of work and family responsibilities, his amygdala was in overdrive. He was living in survival mode. He couldn't get any respite to calmly think through how to bring the knowledge and information he'd gathered about losing weight into his everyday life full of stress.

Wes was like many of my patients. He knew exactly what he had to do but had a hard time putting it into practice because of the many legitimate barriers that existed in his everyday life.

I've found that for most of my patients there's often a gap between knowing something and doing something. My job is to figure out how to close that gap. A lot of the work I do with patients is based on the foundational principles of *motivational interviewing*, which is a technique used in the medical setting to help patients overcome their barriers to change and close the gap. It's a way to meet patients where they are to help them figure out what's most important to them. Three of the most vital elements of motivational interviewing are having empathy, curiosity, and a lack of judgment when understanding how to close the gap between knowing and doing. You can't do motivational interviewing on yourself, because it needs a trained practitioner for it to work. But you can lean into your own empathy, curiosity, and lack of judgment to help you figure out how to close the gap for yourself.

Wes had been ready to take action all along, but he needed my help to devise a realistic plan so he could achieve his goal. My work with Wes was to help him close the gap between knowing what needed to happen and taking action to make it happen.

For Wes's Rule of 2, we focused on his eating habits and weight control, because these were his immediate needs that caused him the most stress. And they addressed what he wanted most—to lose weight.

The first intervention was to encourage Wes to pack a quick and healthy dinner at home to take with him to work. As simple a solution as this seemed, Wes's mornings were so rushed getting the kids ready for school that he didn't think about his own needs until he had already left the house. Because Wes's brain was stressed each morning, it was being led by his amygdala, which focused on his immediate need of getting his kids and himself out the door on time—not on his task of planning and preparing dinner, which was twelve hours in the future. Future planning relies on your prefrontal cortex, which doesn't function optimally when stressed. This is one reason why you're prone to forget simple things like your keys, wallet, or phone during rushed and stressed mornings.

Wes and I devised a plan of his packing dinner for the next day and having it ready to go the night before when he was under less stress. In the morning, he would simply grab it and go, along with his kids.

For our second intervention, instead of Wes speaking to his kids while he sat inside a parked car, we agreed that a better step to reach his weight-loss goal would be for him to get his body moving during the call. He'd video call with his kids from a park with a pond near his office complex. Wes loved fishing and being on the water, so although he couldn't fish every day to relax, a walk near water for twenty minutes was the next best thing. He'd speak to his kids about their day while enjoying the benefits of a city waterscape for himself. He took his kids fishing on weekends, so his daily video call from the pond became an extension of their weekend activity together. Then he would drive to his second job and eat his packed dinner during his first break.

These may seem like simple interventions, but Wes's stress was so high that he was living in self-preservation mode and couldn't think or plan ahead for the next day. He was being guided by his amygdala, not his prefrontal cortex. These two daily interventions, Wes's Rule of 2, helped him get his weight stabilized.

This was a major achievement for Wes. It created a change in his body *and* brain, and caused a ripple effect in his life. His stress improved, along with his energy and motivation. His amygdala was slowly finding its way out of self-preservation mode, and his prefrontal cortex was gaining a stronger foothold. Wes started reviewing his monthly work schedule in advance so he could plan certain days to take longer, thirty-minute walks. With each incremental step, Wes moved closer to his weight-loss goal.

What changed in Wes's mindset to make change possible? He had discovered what mattered to him in the short term and created what I call his MOST goal.

Your Endgame Reveals Your MOST Goal

Discovering what matters most to you is an essential step in making change possible. This is how I've begun nearly every one of my patient visits. The question I ask my patients as they start their journey toward less stress and more resilience is, "What's your endgame? What does 'success' look like to you?"

Sometimes, their answers are immediate and reflexive; at other times a little digging is needed. Over the years, I've heard thousands of responses to these questions, such as:

"I want to have less pain so I can travel through Europe this summer."

"I want my burnout to get better so I have the energy to host Thanksgiving dinner this year."

"I want a job that doesn't make me anxious, but I'm too tired to look for one."

"I want to look good and feel good for my twenty-fifth high school reunion."

"I want to get through cancer therapy and write a children's book."

"I want to have some chaos-free spare time to organize a charity event for my church."

By thinking about what they want, these people were able to start zeroing in on what matters most to them. Knowing what matters most to you is a powerful catalyst for change. Sometimes, it takes a little thought. If you're having trouble coming up with what matters most to you, work on discovering your MOST goal.

TECHNIQUE #1: Uncover Your MOST Goal

We each hold within our minds a mental picture or idea of the best version of ourselves. You're reading this book because you've realized how much unhealthy stress has diverted you from that image. That best-self you envision may seem unattainable at this moment, but that's your stress talking. The resilient you, which is still in there, knows the reason "why" you're ready and willing to change. Your "why" helps tell you what matters most to you in your near future. Once you identify your MOST goal, you will have the clarity and purpose to move forward.

Here are four suggestions to help you craft your MOST goal with the guidelines of being **M**otivating, **O**bjective, **S**mall, and **T**imely:

M: Motivating—Write out a short list of your goals. Then choose one from that list that feels both *motivating* and within reach. Which goal from your list makes you feel energized and fuels you with a sense of motivation? Even if you feel depleted and burned out at the moment, identify the goal that lights you up and offers you a small sliver of hope. Use that as your MOST goal.

O: Objective—*Objective* changes that you can regularly monitor for progress, no matter how tiny or incremental, will help propel you forward through the process of moving toward your MOST goal.

S: Small—Choose a goal that's *small* enough to virtually guarantee your success. Then you can work toward it without many disruptions to your life, and you will feel a sense of real accomplishment.

T: Timely—Choose a goal that's *time-sensitive*. Ideally, you will be able to achieve your MOST goal over the next three months.

If your chosen goal fits within the MOST guidelines, congratulations! You have a guidepost on your way toward less stress and more resilience. Now, write down your MOST goal along with the tentative date three months from now. Mark that date as the official completion of your journey.

From the start, Wes had been clear about his MOST goal, but his sense of overwhelm was a barrier to change. "It feels like there's a long distance between where I want to be and where I am now," he said. At first, packing his dinners just seemed like one more thing to add to his busy schedule. "I mean, I'm used to my drive-thru dinners being easy," he confessed.

Perhaps you can relate to Wes's dilemma. It's easier to keep your daily routine on autopilot, stick to the status quo, and suffer in silence. You can usually keep going for a while, but then one day that canary inside of you is warning of bad things to come. Then, you have no choice but to act.

I assured Wes that it was normal to feel overwhelmed and discouraged about making a change. Change is hard. It's fraught with uncertainty and discomfort, and the human brain is wired to shy away from both. Anticipating discomfort is one of the biggest hurdles to making change possible.[3] Even if you know that change will ultimately help your life in the long run, it's still very hard. "But," I told Wes, "that discomfort you feel when you're doing something new and positive for your stress is a signal of growth."

In one study, people who tolerated a little temporary discomfort while being engaged in different personal growth activities, like writing and educating themselves, were more likely to achieve their goals. The researchers concluded, "Growing is often uncomfortable, but people should seek the discomfort that's inherent in growth as a sign of progress instead of avoiding it."[4]

So being able to tolerate a little temporary discomfort while you're making healthy changes to your life is an indicator that you're stepping into your Growth Zone.

Wes was ready to step into his Growth Zone, beginning with the Rule of 2, only a few lifestyle changes at a time. He had gotten clear about his MOST goal and had accepted that he'd feel a little uncomfortable with his new, positive habits on his way to achieving his goal.

"I have to admit," Wes said, "I really don't know how to start. Where do I begin?"

I handed Wes a blank sheet of paper. "The way to figure that out is to begin with the end in mind," I told him. "We're going to start by creating your Backwards Plan together."

Planning Backwards, Living Forwards

On a blank sheet of paper, I asked Wes to write the word "End" at the top of the paper and next to it to write out his MOST goal and a date about three months in the future. I suggested that he keep the date loose with lots of wiggle room.

At the bottom of the page, I asked Wes to write the word "Start" and put today's date next to the word. Then we worked backwards from the "End," his MOST goal, to the "Start," where he was today. On the line right below his MOST goal, I had Wes write down what would need to happen right before he reached this milestone. For example, Wes wrote: *I'd buy some new pants, in a smaller size, that will look good on me and motivate me to keep going with my weight loss.*

On the line below that one, I had Wes write down what he needed to do to be able to buy new pants. He wrote: *I need to stay on track with my food choices to lose those next two pounds, like I have been doing every week.*

"That's great, Wes," I told him. "Now, keep working backwards. What step do you need to take to lose those next two pounds?"

"I'd stay the course of what is working. I eat the dinner I packed the night before. I even have packed snacks, so I don't use the vending machines at work at all," Wes said, and wrote it down.

"Okay. Move down a line. What's the step to having packed food ready to go?" I asked him.

Wes thought about it for a minute, and then wrote, *When I get home from my night shift, I'm going to listen to this really interesting mystery podcast while I pack up my food and snacks for the next day and get the kids' food ready, too.*

Wes leaned back in his chair, feeling satisfied. "You know, I like what I'm planning. It's a really good podcast, and I never have time to listen to it."

"There you go, Wes. So now we're close to the bottom of the page, the statement of where you are now. What's that first step of where you are now to having your meals packed?"

"Okay. Starting on Saturday morning, the kids will go with me to the grocery store, and we can pick out good food for our lunches and snacks and get enough until next Saturday. Then, we'll go to the store again next week."

"I think you've found a way to start, Wes."

Wes read over his plan one more time.

Using the Backwards Plan, step by step, he realized that his MOST goal was much more within reach than he anticipated. Having a one-page document in his hand, in his own handwriting, helped him feel empowered with his personalized road map to success. It helped him visualize each step in a concrete and tangible way.

TECHNIQUE #2: Make a Backwards Plan

Try this exercise for yourself.

1. At the top of a blank sheet of paper write the word "End," and next to it write down your MOST goal with a date approximately three months into the future.

2. At the bottom of the page, write "Start" and today's date.

3. Now work your way down the page as if you were writing out Google Maps directions in reverse, from the finish to the start. On the line underneath "End," write down the final step you will take right before you reach the "End."

4. Move down another line. Write down the step you will take right before that final step to your goal.

5. Continue to work backwards, figuring out and writing down each step in reverse order. There are no specific number of steps you need to take—only enough to be able to see your Backwards Plan clearly from "End" (achieving your MOST goal) to "Start" (today).

When you make it stepwise down to your "Start," you have a complete list of directions to follow, step-by-step.

Your Backwards Plan is a visual representation of your journey in real time. As most great athletes will tell you, if you can see it, then you can be it. Your Backwards Plan helps you overcome the biggest hurdle of change: taking that first step forward into action.

When Wes came to see me two months later, he showed me his Backwards Plan. He'd made it more than halfway through; he had already lost fourteen pounds, and his destination was closer than ever.

"I have to confess, I had a setback for three days," Wes told me. "It was my work buddy's birthday, and we went out and had onion rings, milk shakes, and double burgers. It was so good I went to that burger joint the next two nights on my own. I was so mad at myself after the second night. Then, I went ahead and had it again the next night."

"It's okay, Wes," I said. "We feel peer pressure sometimes. I'm sure your work buddy is used to your past routine of eating burgers and fries."

"He is. And I didn't want to explain my Rule of 2 to him in case I failed. Then I made myself fail the next two nights."

"It looks like you turned it back around, though. Our efforts at resetting an old pattern can be on a sliding scale, Wes. That's where some compassion for yourself can really help," I said. "I'd like to know what made you go back to your MOST goal?"

"I wish I could tell you that I didn't want to let you or myself down," Wes said with a shy smile. "But the truth is, this really great single woman who manages the grocery store where the kids and I shop told me I was looking better and better all the time."

I started to laugh and so did Wes.

"Hmm, it seems like change isn't that hard after all," I said.

There's nothing better than witnessing patients like Wes experience a whole new level of happiness from working toward and then reaching their MOST goals.

Reaching for Happiness

If I were to ask you a big question like "What do you want out of life?" you would probably say, "I want to be happy." In fact, "how to be happy" has been one of Google's most searched terms for the past five years and had its greatest popularity in 2020 when the world was in lockdown. Makes sense, right? Happiness is a seriously coveted goal, not just for my patients, but for most people around the world.

Happiness doesn't help you get any closer to your "why" because happiness is a vague and moving target. We all want to be happy; it's a universal yearning shared by every human being on the planet, but research has shown that we're not very good at predicting what's going to make us happy.[5] For this reason, it's important for you to get very specific about your endgame and MOST goal and those all-important steps of your Backwards Plan. They are concrete and tangible, whereas happiness isn't.

Ryan was a thirty-six-year-old music executive who visited me for uncontrolled anxiety. He worked in the music industry with some of the biggest performers in the business. There was no question that Ryan had a life that many people would envy. He owned three condos—one in Manhattan, one in Aspen, and one in Paris. He spent summer months on a yacht in the Mediterranean and winters in Aspen. He had worked hard to achieve this level of success, but now he often suffered from crippling anxiety.

"You would think I'd feel great about where I'm at and being able to afford almost anything I want, but I don't," Ryan told me during his first office visit. "I feel like I'm shaking from the inside out. I pace the floor almost every night, all night long. Sometimes my arms and my lips feel like they're tingling. I can't even read a book because my anxiety is so bad." Ryan was seeing a psychiatrist for medications, along with a therapist.

"They're the only two people I don't feel afraid to talk to. I used to be the most social guy in the room. Not anymore. I duck out of the backstage door as soon as I possibly can to avoid having to meet and talk to new people."

He had entered his profession with a clear sense of purpose. He loved music and felt a deep connection to the musical community. At the start of his career, he craved the perks that went hand in hand with his job: the parties, designer clothes, cars, cash, and high-end restaurants; the spoils of a luxury lifestyle. But after ten years in the business, the hectic travel schedule and constant jet lag were taking their toll on his health. He was starting to despise his job, and he longed to quit the industry. He felt numb about his success and was eager to make a change.

After listening to his story, I asked Ryan what had made him happy before his current career.

"I have no idea," Ryan said. "I barely remember my life before this career."

"Then go back to before you were old enough to seek out a career," I suggested. "What was the thing you looked forward to doing when you were a kid or a teenager?"

For the first time during our visit, Ryan smiled. "My best days were with my grandfather. He was in really great shape, even in his seventies. I'd spend the weekend with him in New Hampshire, and he and I would hike in the White Mountains."

As Ryan was recalling the experience, his face and shoulders relaxed, and his breathing slowed down. "Those were great times," he continued. "We'd pick a steep trail, climb to the high point, and sit and talk. We'd watch the hawks and sometimes see an eagle. I even liked the days when it rained. Then, at night we'd build a fire pit in my grandpa's backyard, and I'd play my guitar for him."

"Do you still play guitar?" I asked him.

"Not in about a decade. It's bizarre. Playing guitar is what made me totally want a career in the music industry," he said. "Now, I never pick one up."

"Did you lose interest?"

"No, I miss it. And I miss my grandfather. He died about four years ago. I bought a condo in Aspen in his memory, but it's not the same."

"I'm sorry to hear about your grandfather, but you still have your guitar, right? And, there are mountains where you can still hike, if you want."

Ryan nodded, already knowing where I was going.

Before he left my office, we set up a plan for how Ryan could reset his stress and burnout. I suggested he begin the Rule of 2 with the activities that he loved most.

Ryan committed to playing his guitar for at least twenty minutes every day for the pure joy of playing. He didn't have to perform for anyone or even sound good. The goal was to experience how much he loved music.

Although his work travel didn't always put him close to a hiking trail, he committed to getting out in nature in some way every single day, and taking a walk. I wanted him to take in the sky, the trees, or whatever form of nature might be around him, even if it was merely in a couple of brisk loops around city blocks.

I didn't see Ryan again for four months, but we kept in touch through email. After the first two months, he sent a positive update. He had reconfigured his work schedule to travel less than before. He was spending longer stretches of time in his home in Aspen to be near the mountains. He had recently joined a mountaineering club; the man running the club reminded him of his grandfather. He also played his guitar every day and was considering joining a guitar collective in town.

Reorienting his life to pursue more intrinsically rewarding experiences rather than externally validating experiences helped Ryan reset his stress, which had a ripple effect on his sleep and anxiety. The sum of these changes was a balm to his nervous system.

When I saw Ryan in person several months later, it was apparent that he was becoming a changed man.

He felt calm, purposeful, and grounded. His anxiety was much better controlled. His psychiatrist was even considering tapering his medication dosage under supervision because he was doing so well, much better than he had in years.

In four months, Ryan had reset his brain and body and was getting his anxiety in check.

Ryan had many material comforts at his disposal, yet he still found himself stuck in self-preservation mode without a way out. So perhaps you're wondering, "Why didn't he figure it out for himself and make a quick pivot? How did he still get so far off track?"

The changes he made were small, simple strategies that he could've done anywhere, anytime—playing guitar daily and hiking—but because his amygdala was working in overdrive, it was hard for him to get out of his own way.

When it comes to you and your life, why does change for the better seem to be such an effort instead of something you do simply because it feels good and makes you feel happier? It turns out, there are two kinds of happiness, and each one affects your brain and body in distinctly different ways. Happiness is a complicated construct that uses many different brain areas, but one kind is more lasting than the other, and Ryan was chasing the kind of happiness that doesn't last.

Two Kinds of Happiness

The first kind of happiness is called *hedonic happiness*. This was the kind of happiness—centered around pleasure and consumption—that Ryan had initially filled his life with. Delicious meals, tropical vacations, and Netflix binges are all modern-day examples of hedonic happiness. It's not necessarily about the cost of an item; it's about how it makes you feel.

When you participate in hedonic activities, like treating yourself to an extra large coffee with whipped cream, splurging on the latest electronic device, or buying yourself a new pair of shoes, you're giving your brain and body a gift. During these moments, your brain is flooded with dopamine, the pleasure hormone, and you feel an instantaneous rush of joy throughout your body. This kind of happiness is very real to your brain. It's intended to serve an important purpose: it gives your brain and body a brief, but necessary, respite from the routines of everyday life. Allowing yourself occasional opportunities for hedonic happiness can serve as a temporary release valve to slow down the tea kettle scenario of stress. But in the same way that stress can be healthy or unhealthy depending on the dose and frequency, the same applies to hedonic happiness.

In small doses, hedonic happiness serves an important and vital role for your psychological well-being. But in larger and more frequent doses, it loses its appeal to your brain and body. You can't depend on hedonic happiness as your primary source of happiness, as Ryan did, precisely because its effects are fleeting and short-lived. By its very nature, hedonic happiness is designed to leave you wanting more. This phenomenon is called the *hedonic treadmill*.[6]

Scientists believe that we each have a distinct set point for how much hedonic happiness we can experience. It's called a treadmill because, except for the initial jolt of joy you get from any hedonic activity, your brain will eventually return to its baseline level of happiness. You can chase the high of hedonic happiness, but you can't make it last.

One woman, Debra, described it like this: "When I've had a tough week at work, I'll stop at a Louis Vuitton or Gucci store and find a bag that I love. The sales clerks are always enthusiastic and really pay attention to me. Everything is beautiful in the shop, so it's fun to be there. Then they box up my new bag like a special gift, put it in an elegant shopping bag, and I carry it out. I'm in heaven. However, a couple of weeks later, after the compliments on my new purchase from co-workers are over, my happy buzz ends and the bag becomes just one more purse in my closet. My stress at work hasn't changed at all, and the stress of my next credit card bill piles it on even more."

The hedonic treadmill can take many forms. The third piece of cake isn't as pleasurable as the first, for example, or pursuing a new love interest loses its thrill. Hedonic pleasures become less exciting over time, because the initial dopamine surge levels off in your brain. You're left back where you started. You can get hooked by craving more and more of the same, or you begin to seek out novelty, to feel another jolt of instantaneous joy.

This isn't a design flaw of your brain. Your brain's hedonic treadmill is actually a protective mechanism. Studies show that even if people have wonderful or tragic experiences, they eventually return to their set point of happiness.[7] Irrespective of the quality of your external experiences, positive or negative, hedonic happiness helps you cope temporarily in the moment by opening the steam valve on your tea kettle of stress.

After a long day of meetings, speaking to a large group, parenting, and even while writing this book, I've craved a good two-hour Netflix binge. Even with very limited personal time, some online retail therapy will give me a dopamine rush. And a spa day is my favorite hedonic fallback. These positive moments can serve as circuit breakers and are fantastic when my stress response is haywire. But without question, they are only temporary fixes that do very little to rewire the brain for less stress in the long run.

We can't rely solely on hedonic experiences to cure our stress, because the hedonic treadmill is always running in the background. To cure our stress for the long term, we have to learn how to work with our biology. That's when a new and different kind of happiness comes in. It's called *eudaimonic happiness,* and it's the gateway for curing our unhealthy stress for good.[8]

"I got approached, as a landscape designer, to help plan out a community city garden," I heard from Kevin. "It was a project for low-income families to grow vegetables on a lot where an old building had been demolished. Even though I've designed green spaces for high-end office buildings, this community garden project has really been satisfying for me. When I'm there, putting the plans in motion, helping the kids plant bell peppers, I never even look at my phone or think about what time it is. It's a lot of work, but I feel happier than ever. And the unexpected bonus is, my doctor says my blood pressure has gone down!"

Eudaimonic happiness isn't centered on pleasure and joy, like hedonic happiness is—it's centered on meaning and purpose. Humans are meaning-seeking, purpose-driven creatures, which makes this kind of happiness the pot of gold on our stress journey. We can keep leveling up on experiences that create meaning and purpose without worrying that the effects will be fleeting or short-lived because there is no eudaimonic treadmill.

You've had many eudaimonic experiences in your life, you just haven't called them that. Think of the experiences that created a feeling of calm contentment. They are the activities that in the long run become growth-oriented. Eudaimonic experiences give you a sense of belonging, community, connection, and altruism. Donating your time for a cause, gardening, learning to play an instrument, painting, cooking meals at a mission, or building a wheelchair ramp for a neighbor are just a few examples of what may provide a eudaimonically happy experience.

Because meaning and purpose are central to eudaimonic happiness and also highly individualized, your idea of what makes you eudaimonically happy will be different from someone else's. Regardless of the mode to eudaimonic happiness, once you tap into your sense of meaning and purpose, your brain and body recognize what's happening and respond accordingly in some remarkable ways.

In one study, eighty people were assessed for "hedonic and eudaimonic well-being."[9] Researchers looked at the genomes, the coding within our DNA, of these people and found stark differences in genetic expression. Eudaimonic well-being was linked to a stronger antiviral and antibody response and lower levels of inflammatory markers, whereas higher levels of hedonic well-being had the opposite effect. For the purposes of this discussion, the lower the level of inflammatory markers, the better. This was the first study to show genetic differences in the two kinds of happiness. The key takeaway? Not all happiness is created equal!

According to the researchers, "Doing good and feeling good have very different effects on the human genome . . . Apparently, the human genome is much more sensitive to different ways of achieving happiness than are conscious minds."[10]

As clearly seen by this study, our bodies are very good at telling the difference between the two kinds of happiness. The conundrum is that we as people aren't as good at it!

What Makes Us Happy?

In spite of how much thought and time we all spend trying to achieve happiness, we're actually pretty bad at figuring out what makes us happy. I asked Dr. Laurie Santos, professor of psychology at Yale University and the host of *The Happiness Lab* podcast, about why this happens.

"If you ask people what they think a truly happy life would be . . . [it might be] lying on the beach and eating ice cream, something with no stress whatsoever. People have misconceptions when it comes to stress and happiness. A little bit of stress is a good thing," Santos offered.

As we've discussed already, stress is a necessary part of your healthy functioning biology. As it turns out, stress is also important for your happiness.

"Happiness is multifaceted," Santos continued. "A sense of meaning contributes to your satisfaction . . . because you're doing things that are meaningful [to you]. That feels good because you're in flow."

The state of *flow*, a term originally coined by psychologist Mihaly Csikszentmihalyi, is when you are fully immersed in an activity and there's a sense of ease, mastery, enjoyment, and timelessness.

"People don't necessarily think of flow when they're going for leisure after they've had a tough week at work." Santos said. I can understand that. After a long week at work, I want to do the easiest thing possible, like ordering takeout and binge-watching a series on a streaming service. I know that it won't provide long-lasting happiness, but it does provide short-lived satisfaction in the moment, which is what I sometimes need after a long and difficult work week. Hedonic experiences have a legitimate and valuable role as temporary circuit breakers for your stress. Distraction is a viable coping strategy for stress after a hard day's work, and hedonic experiences are wonderful distractions when needed. You just can't rely only on them for sustainable happiness over time.

Santos also says that our intuitions about leisure aren't always accurate. The easy, leisurely path filled with hedonic experiences can quickly get boring and lose appeal, as it eventually did for Ryan. Ultimately, engaging in leisure activities that involve a bit more of a challenge for your brain can help you create the state of flow, which then can lead to more substantial, long-lasting happiness.

Realistically, it's ideal to strike a balance between seeking hedonic experiences for short-term gratification along with eudaimonic experiences for long-term meaning and purpose. Both types of happiness add value to your life, but only one has sustainable benefits for your brain and body. Sometimes, when you've been running fast on your hedonic treadmill, it can take an unexpected crisis to reassess what matters most in your life.

Carmen was referred to me by her oncologist because she had recently been diagnosed with stage 4 ovarian cancer. Her oncologist had been forthright about her terminal prognosis, but he was willing to try an experimental therapy to possibly slow down the cancer's rapid progression. Carmen was a sixty-two-year-old lawyer. She worked long hours for many years. Her work was intense, and she frequently oversaw several cases at a time.

"I always told myself that when I was closer to retirement age, I would scale back my work hours," she explained to me in my office one mild April afternoon. "But the opposite happened. More and more clients needed me. I ended up working more hours than ever before."

She paused to look at me, to see whether I understood. I did. We are both in the business of helping people in trouble. It's very hard to turn people away. I empathized with Carmen.

When she was diagnosed with cancer, she tried to continue working on her stack of cases through the course of her treatments, to "stay distracted," but eventually it got to be too much for her. She had to give up her job.

She almost seemed apologetic for stepping away from work. "I'm not a quitter. I would've worked until I was eighty if I could."

"Do you miss it? Did you enjoy your work?" I asked.

Her answer surprised me.

"Not really. I used to love it when I was younger. But I haven't enjoyed it at all for the past decade or so."

Carmen had been born into poverty and had, in her words, "made it out." She was proud of her accomplishments. She had educated herself and built her career so that she could provide a secure life for herself and her family.

"I've never taken anything I have for granted, but this diagnosis has really sidelined me," she said. "It's made me question everything."

Carmen was eager for a reset. "Without my job, I don't really know how to act anymore. If I can't say 'I'm a lawyer,' then who am I? I don't want to be known as only a person going through cancer treatments. There must be something else."

"We'll work on finding your something else together. What if you consider this time in your life as an open door to do the things that bring you joy?" I asked.

"There's a good thought. I like that idea," Carmen said.

"What are the things that bring you happiness?"

Carmen was stumped. "It's been a long time since I asked myself what I want to do because it brings me joy. I'm always doing things for everyone else—my family, my clients, my community. It's never about me."

I read a quotation attributed to Carl Jung and asked her to reflect on it: "What did you do as a child that made the hours pass like minutes? Herein lies the secret to your earthly pursuits."

Carmen's face lit up. "I used to love making things with my hands as a kid. I could spend hours making clay people. My sister and I would play with them on the front stoop of our house all afternoon. It was my own little world and it brought me so much joy."

Then she said, "In fact, where I currently live, I think I bought my house because its front stoop reminds me of those happy afternoons as a kid. We would even sit out there to do our homework. I have great wicker furniture on my stoop now, but I only walk by it. I never take the time to sit and watch the world go by."

"Let's start there!" I said.

I suggested she use the Rule of 2 to focus on two things she could do when she left my office to cultivate her sense of eudaimonic happiness. I wanted her to do these activities for the sake of joy, without the need for external validation or praise.

"Let's add two things to your routine that bring you joy. So today on your way home, stop by an art store and pick up some clay. Start by making one sculpture at least once a week for the next month. Don't judge yourself as you do it. You're not showing it to anyone, it's just for you.

"And the second thing you're going to do," I continued, "is spend time making use of those wicker chairs on your stoop, for at least thirty minutes a couple times a week while the weather's warm. That's your Rule of 2 for the next month."

"That's my prescription? Sitting on my stoop? Doing nothing?" Carmen asked me incredulously.

"You can read or write or do whatever you want to do," I said. "But I think doing nothing but watching the world go by is a great use of time."

"It sounds like heaven," Carmen said.

The starting point with Carmen seemed clear because of the sheer delight on her face when she was thinking of her childhood joys.

Carmen was also working with a skilled team of physicians and psychologists to manage the fundamental aspects of her care, such as sleep, appetite, and coping. Our visits together were an added layer. My job was to support Carmen on her healing journey.

There's a difference between being healed and being cured. If you have a disease that can't be cured, you can still be healed. Healing is movement in the direction of positive results, releasing negative patterns and emotions, and can also feel mentally and emotionally therapeutic beyond your physical diagnosis. Regardless of how Carmen's cancer diagnosis went, my work with her was to help her heal.

Creating a warm, connected, and therapeutic relationship with a patient isn't just a nice gesture; it can positively influence health outcomes. Studies show that doctors who offer support, reassurance, and kindness can help their patients' discomfort and symptoms. "The simple things a doctor says and does to connect with patients can make a difference for health outcomes," write two researchers in psychology.[11] From a medical standpoint, Carmen was unlikely to be cured from her advanced stage of aggressive cancer. But our work together could help her decrease stress and create meaning and purpose during the difficult and often demoralizing treatment process.[12] Whether or not you're facing a health struggle like Carmen, it's helpful to find doctors who make you feel like you've had a therapeutic encounter with them.

When I saw Carmen for her follow-up four weeks later, I was wowed by her progress. She had committed to the Rule of 2 in a big way! She had immersed herself in her clay sculptures and created a small art workspace in her home for her ongoing projects. She brought me photos of her work, and I could see that she had some serious talent. She also sat on her stoop for thirty minutes almost every day. She said these two activities brought her so much joy.

I continued to see Carmen every month throughout her healing journey. Her sculptures got larger and more intricate. She told me how one of her friends wanted to have a gallery show of her work because it was so good, and she was considering it—but only if she wanted to. When I asked her how she was feeling, she said, "I haven't been this content and fulfilled in a long time." And then she joked, "All it took was a cancer diagnosis to get me here!"

As the months passed, Carmen kept going with her Rule of 2. I've had many patients like Carmen, over my years in practice, who've made radical changes in their lives when faced with the wake-up call of a terminal diagnosis. Usually, they're changes the person had already planned to make but then put off or set aside for so many reasons.

I've often wondered why it takes something as dire as a terminal diagnosis to make us take stock of what our lives have become. Isn't there a kinder and gentler way to figure out what matters most?

I'm here to tell you that you can find more eudaimonic happiness starting today. It's something you deserve to do for yourself, every single day. There's no need to wait for a crisis. In fact, figuring out your own eudaimonic happiness now might prevent a more difficult wake-up call down the road.

Here's where your canary can help you. For many of my patients, they often describe a distinct moment of time when they have a personal revelation about what needs to change. But it's not like in the movies on a beautiful trip where you reach a sunny meadow and reflect on your life. It's usually a moment that blindsides you on a Tuesday afternoon. You get so fed up with the status quo that you're desperate for a change. Your canary's song is impossible to ignore. That moment for me was 10 p.m. every night with the stampede of horses. What was it for you?

TECHNIQUE #3: Find Your Buried Treasure

1. Without censoring yourself, write down five activities you did in the past or as a child that brought you joy and made the hours pass like minutes.

2. Pick one or two of those activities that you could begin incorporating into your life starting tomorrow.

3. Organize the materials you'll need for the activity: pens and paints, a musical instrument, a pair of sneakers, a model kit, some gardening tools, or a bike? Chances are you still have them somewhere in your house.

4. Commit to doing one activity for at least ten or twenty minutes every day, even if it's only riding up and down the street on your bike, doodling on a pad of paper, filling flower pots with soil, or playing scales on an instrument. Even five minutes a day can make a difference. No amount of time or effort is too little to have a positive effect on your brain.

5. Put a checkmark on a calendar every day that you do the activity. Even if life gets busy, try not to break your streak of checkmarks. If you skip a few days, it's okay. It may have been a long time since you allowed yourself to have pure fun. Let yourself start again.

6. Congratulate yourself for every day that you give yourself a checkmark! It's a day that you're doing something positive for your brain. You're slowly rewiring your brain for more lasting happiness.

The Power of Possibility

Now that you've crystallized your "why" and defined what your end-game is and what matters MOST to you, allow yourself to feel the possibility of it coming true. Not necessarily right now, which may not feel authentic, but the possibility of it happening sometime in the near future because it's within your reach and closer than you think.

Why bother to feel the possibility? Because it's a way to activate the laws of physics, which help to prime our brains and bodies for change. Not to get too technical, but there are two types of energy in physics: kinetic energy and potential energy. Kinetic energy is active movement, and potential energy is dormant inertia. According to Isaac Newton, energy can't be created or destroyed; it can only change forms from potential to kinetic or vice versa. When we let ourselves zoom out to consider the possibility of our MOST goal coming true, we start to wake up that dormant potential energy from its status quo state so that it can become the kinetic energy of change.

Harnessing the power of possibility is actually used in real-world achievements all the time, especially when the stakes are high, like in professional sports. There is perhaps no better segment of the population that relies on the power of the mind-body connection than professional athletes. Athletes inherently know that their mental game out of the arena is just as valuable as their physical game in the arena. Sports psychologists are an integral part of any training regimen because they help players rewire their brains to visualize success. Legendary basketball star Michael Jordan, tennis champion Serena Williams, Olympic gold medal swimmer Michael Phelps, and many other elite athletes have reported using the power of visualization to achieve great results.[13] Perhaps visualization can help you achieve your own brand of greatness too.

It's also perfectly okay if you don't feel very changeable right now or if you're skeptical about whether you'll really be able to rewire your brain and body for less stress and more resilience. Trust the physics of the process anyway. Skepticism is a healthy and normal part of this process. I love my skeptical patients because when change does inevitably happen, they're often the most enthusiastic. In science-speak, they've increased their sense of self-efficacy, or the belief that they have the ability to make change happen for themselves. That's why

I'm asking you to start small, to build confidence in your self-efficacy, and know that you have the power to change your energy from inertia to action.

An example of small steps leading to greater self-efficacy is one Dr. Edward Phillips shared with me: One of his patients was reluctant to walk but agreed to walk with her friend twice per week. After a couple of weeks of consistent walking, she came to see him again with a smile on her face. "I know I said I was going to walk twice per week. But I didn't do what we agreed. I love seeing my friend and the weather is getting better. So I'm walking five days a week!"

"Our bodies are wonderfully adaptable, that's just basic physiology" says Phillips. "We're also psychologically adaptable and we yearn to get better. I think, inherently, people *want* to get better."

More and more, in our modern-day lives, we don't meet the challenge of managing stress and burnout because we don't take stock of exactly what's consuming our time and attention. If we knew better, we could do better. I know many of my patients are surprised to learn that something they use every day and all day long has been a big contributor to their stress. When they learn about this hidden source of continual stress, which we'll talk about in the next chapter, they realize they have endless opportunities throughout their day to practice and perfect their self-efficacy.

As you now know, the First Reset is about identifying and making a plan toward less stress, while at the same time giving you something to look forward to every day. Like Wes, you chose a reasonable MOST goal, something that you knew would make you feel a sense of motivation and then accomplishment within a three-month time frame. Once you had that MOST goal, you could visualize it coming to fruition step-by-step by using the Backwards Plan technique. Finally, as you progress to your three-month MOST goal, you can offset stress daily by Finding Your Buried Treasure in the same way Ryan and Carmen did. This simple pleasure that you may have long set aside will help you cultivate the lasting benefit of eudaimonic happiness.

This First Reset and the techniques within lay the foundation for the overall upgrade to more resilience and far less stress that's available to you now. So let's keep moving forward together. In the Second Reset, you'll learn how to find quiet in this noisy world, protect your mental bandwidth, and finally get the rest and recovery your brain and body deserve.

4

The Second Reset: Find Quiet in a Noisy World

A message was taped to my office door when I got back from a staff meeting. A former patient, Nicole, had stopped by looking for me. She wrote that she had to tell me about something that had happened to her.

She and I had worked closely the previous year for about five months to help her with her high stress and what she called "my ADHD." She had seen a psychiatrist who had reassured her she didn't have a diagnosis of attention-deficit/hyperactivity disorder, but she told me she was unable to finish projects and was always distracted. She wanted to learn how to manage her stress so she could improve her focus over longer periods of time.

We had applied the Rule of 2, and Nicole was seeing incredible improvements in her ability to concentrate. She was working to find quiet in a noisy world.

I called her during my next break, with a bit of trepidation that something was causing her acute stress.

"You're not going to believe this when I tell you," Nicole said, her voice spilling over with laughter.

I breathed a sigh of relief. I could hear the enthusiasm in her voice. She sounded much better than when she was struggling with stress.

"What's going on?"

"Two hours! I went two whole hours without checking it once!" Nicole told me. "In fact, I didn't even open the desk drawer it was in. I had to share this unbelievable milestone with you." At this point, I started to laugh too. I knew exactly what "it" was: her smartphone.

The most detrimental relationship in your life is most likely the thing glowing in the palm of your hand: your smartphone. Research shows that your relationship with your phone has a great impact on your level of stress and consumes most of your attention and mental bandwidth, much more than your relationship with your partner or kids or even your extended family and work colleagues. You may perceive your smartphone as harmless and relaxing, a respite from the daily grind, but it actually has the opposite effect. It's blatantly rewiring your brain for more stress. Recent statistics show that almost half of us spend five to six hours a day on our phones, and we physically touch our phones about 2,617 times a day![1]

Smartphones aren't the only source of digital noise causing stress in our lives: screens of all kinds, including cable TV, tablets, and computers, also steal our mental energy and attention. Most of us know that spending too much time on these devices is "bad" for us, but as a doctor I can tell you that they have a bigger impact on our brains, stress levels, and even our overall well-being than we realize.

The Second Reset, Finding Quiet in a Noisy World, will help you create practical and actionable boundaries around these digital distractions that add to your unhealthy stress, and teach you some new techniques for getting the deep, restorative sleep your unhealthy stress may have taken from you. Through no fault of your own, as an informed citizen of the modern world, you've been shortchanging your brain's capacity for rest and recovery without realizing it. The techniques in this Second Reset will help you get back the rest and recovery your brain needs.

Nicole's news about not checking her phone for several hours was a huge leap forward for her. When I had met her, she never let it out of her sight. In fact, at one time it was the most important relationship in her life. And Nicole isn't alone in this all-consuming bond; most of us have the same infatuation. Yet she was able to change her pattern and was thrilled with her newfound ability to focus on a work project for two hours without ever scrolling on her phone. What a change for someone who admittedly checked her phone dozens of times in one hour. Nicole's experience proves that all of us are capable of changing our relationship with our digital distractors—because we all deserve to find our quiet in a noisy world.

As Nicole had figured out through the Rule of 2, where your attention goes, your energy and mental bandwidth soon follow.

What is your mental bandwidth? Your bandwidth is your brain's ability to focus, learn new ideas, make decisions, and stay on track. It's your attention, and at any moment there are endless external forces vying for it.

You might be thinking, "What's the big deal? Everybody texts and checks email and social media on their phones. That's how life is now." But despite the many technological advances for speed and efficiency in your life, your mental bandwidth has distinctly human limitations. It's not an infinite resource in ample supply. In the same way your body gets physically tired from overexertion, your brain can get exhausted, too.

Like me, you may be experiencing the constant push and pull of competing priorities: work pressures, family obligations, health concerns, and even making time to pursue your personal interests. It's easy to feel stretched thin. How can you make inroads in your stress struggle when you feel like your bandwidth is used up? There's only one way. Create boundaries around your most valuable resource: your attention.

Designing Your Digital Boundaries

Our reliance on our phones has been correlated with worsening stress-related conditions, mood disorders, sleep disorders, increased irritability, hypervigilance, anxiety, poor concentration, and difficulty completing complex tasks. And that's just when you're using your phone. Studies also show that the mere presence of a phone nearby, even when not in use, can decrease your brainpower through a phenomenon known as *brain drain* because of its sheer potential for distraction.[2]

It turns out that this small, inanimate object you hold in the palm of your hand has some pretty big consequences on your attention, brain health, and stress. The only way to curb its effect on you is to design a boundary around your dependence on it. The goal of the Second Reset isn't to make you relinquish your phone, which is both unrealistic and unnecessary from the scientific point of view. One study of 619 people found that decreasing their smartphone use, rather than total abstinence, led to better well-being and more sustainable mental health outcomes.[3]

Therefore, I wouldn't ask you to become a digital monk, renounce technology, and live an analog life. Technology can be a wonderful thing, helping us stay informed, connected, and engaged. And with artificial intelligence being brought into many industries, technology is an important part of modern life. However, awareness of its potential to steal your mental bandwidth is essential for stress relief and burnout recovery.

The Second Reset, Finding Quiet in a Noisy World, isn't about a breakup with your smartphone. Like I suggest to many of my patients, it's time to *reconsider* your relationship to your phone. It's about being in control of your phone instead of your phone controlling what you think about and how you feel all day long. I want to teach you how to create a healthy boundary around your attention so you can redirect it to what matters most on your journey to less stress. Think of me as your relationship coach.

You may not be convinced that your relationship with your phone is affecting your stress. Most of my patients initially don't understand the connection. They see their smartphones as a convenience that makes their lives easier. And in many ways, that's true. We don't have to pull over in the car to use a pay phone anymore. We can get messages to family members and friends in a flash. We can get driving directions within seconds and no one has to spread a map out on the dashboard of the car and try to figure out which way is north or south. Who doesn't appreciate all of that and more about having a smartphone? However, most of us don't use our smartphones only when we need them; we become attached to them in an unhealthy way—using them all day and sometimes all night too.

Here's a simple way to gauge your own mental reliance on your smartphone. Keep a piece of paper and pen right next to you for three or four hours. Whenever you feel the impulse to check your phone, put a tally mark on the paper. Even if you don't actually pick up your phone, try to honestly make a mark for every time the thought of looking at your phone comes to mind. Most of my patients and friends have been astounded by the number of tally marks on the paper.

One friend even joked with a nervous laugh, “Unbelievable! I filled up the front of the paper and had to flip it over and use the back, too. I know we take about 960 breaths per hour. It’s almost as if I wanted to check my phone every time I took a breath in! Help!”

I’m here to help without judgment, because I’m not in a position to critique my friend or anyone else. Trust me, I’m right there with you. I know all the science about stress and media use, and I still feel compelled to check my phone multiple times an hour. Those little devices have a lot of pull on our mental bandwidth.

When I noticed this phenomenon play out with my patients, it seemed clear to me that asking them about media use and their mental reliance on smartphones needed to be part of my standard protocol for clinical decision-making. I’ve witnessed firsthand just how profoundly technology can influence our stress pathway with many of my patients.

Julian was one such patient. He came to see me for medically unexplained fatigue after his primary care doctor did a full workup but found nothing abnormal with blood tests and cardiac imaging. Julian’s fatigue had gotten so bad that it was interfering with his work as a public transportation train conductor. He was fed up and exhausted when he came to see me. His fatigue was affecting his mood and his quality of life.

Julian had always loved his job, but for the first time in seventeen years, he was too exhausted to get through his shifts. He had started squeezing in frequent naps in the break room whenever he had the chance. He had usually been the person who could be counted on to pick up extra shifts, but that was no longer possible. In fact, he was starting to scale back on his work hours because of his fatigue.

He had noticed personality changes too. He described himself as “happy-go-lucky” and “mellow,” but over the previous few months he had been feeling irritable and quick to anger. "It's like I'm always waiting for the other shoe to drop," he said. "I'm just not sure why I feel so on edge."

I asked him what he did during his time away from work. "I'm a newsie," he told me proudly. "I can tell you what's going on almost anywhere in the world."

When I asked him how closely he followed breaking news and current events, he replied, "Whenever I'm home and awake—and sometimes when I'm sleeping too."

I laughed, thinking it was a joke. But Julian wasn't joking.

He started his day at 6 a.m. He would pick up his phone from his nightstand and start reading the news headlines before he got up out of bed. He then would scroll through social media while eating breakfast and watch a little TV in his bedroom as he got dressed for work. During breaks at work, he'd read through headlines. At lunch, he would do the same. When he got home, he'd make dinner with a news channel on in the background and eat while scrolling again through social media on his phone. He'd wind down at night in front of the twenty-four-hour news channels until he fell asleep.

"Over the past few years, I've felt really bothered by what's going on in the news," Julian told me. "I watch and read more and then end up staying up later than I'd like to almost every night. A lot of nights, I'll fall asleep on the couch and wake up hours later with the TV still on."

He hadn't planned on leaving the TV on overnight, but it became a habit, and now he couldn't stay asleep unless the TV was on. So Julian wasn't kidding when he said he consumed media when he was awake and sometimes while he was sleeping!

He had been at a friend's barbecue recently, and a couple of his buddies started to good-naturedly tease him about looking at his phone constantly. One even joked whether Julian may have missed his calling as a news anchor.

"Do you think your friends are onto something?" I asked him.

"My friends know that I'm a newsie," Julian said. "They obviously don't think about how bad things are in the world right now. It's a complete shitshow. Something new every minute. It's hard to keep up, but I try to stay informed."

"Maybe they just don't need to know what's going on every minute," I suggested. "From your story, it seems like they may feel you're not really present with them when you spend time with them."

"Sure. Maybe. I can definitely see that," Julian said, while at the same time taking a quick glance at a breaking news alert that popped up on his phone's home screen. Then he looked up at me with a sheepish grin and said, "Okay, I guess it's gotten out of hand."

Julian's fatigue, sleep problems, and mood changes correlated perfectly with his uptick in media use. I suggested there could be a link, and he raised his eyebrows skeptically. He wasn't convinced that his media use could lead to his symptoms. "Come on! Do you really think my phone and my TV are messing me up? Everybody does this now!"

Julian was right. We're attached to our devices more than ever. Everywhere we go, in any line, in any waiting room, in the afterschool pick-up lane, even waiting for the walk signal to cross a busy street, we take that moment to check our phones. If we have an idle moment, chances are we're looking at our phone screen. It doesn't even have to be downtime. In Boston, where I live, I routinely see pedestrians crossing busy city streets during rush hour with their eyes glued to their screens, day and night. Near-miss injuries to distracted pedestrians who are looking at their phone screens instead of their surroundings are now considered a growing public safety issue.[4]

A Classic Case of Popcorn Brain

Julian was suffering from an increasingly common condition known as *popcorn brain*. While not a true medical diagnosis, popcorn brain is a growing cultural phenomenon. It's a term coined by researcher David Levy to describe what happens to our brains when we spend too much time online.[5] Our brain circuitry starts to "pop" from being overstimulated by the fast-paced information stream. Over time, our brains get habituated to this constant streaming of information, making it harder for us to look away and disconnect from our devices, slow down our thoughts, and live fully *offline*, where things move at a much different, and slower, pace.[6] What makes popcorn brain so difficult to identify is that it's ubiquitous and, as Julian correctly pointed out, increasingly becoming the norm. In fact, 85 percent of American adults go online daily, and three in ten describe themselves as "constantly online."[7]

We are all at risk of developing popcorn brain when we overconsume media. Maybe you're not interested in the news like Julian was; maybe you prefer social media instead. One of my patients was concerned that he had an "Instagram addiction" because he checked Instagram on his phone every fifteen minutes. Another patient who works as a social media influencer was waking up nearly every hour throughout the night to monitor and track the metrics of engagement on her posts. Just as there are many manifestations of maladaptive stress, there are also many manifestations of popcorn brain, each with its own flavor.

For Julian, his exhaustion, irritability, and fatigue were telltale signs of his popcorn brain. He was fed up with feeling exhausted and very concerned that he might cause an injury by being so tired at work. He agreed to follow my suggested Rule of 2 for sixty days, with zero expectations. He left my office with two courses of action to follow.

The Media Diet

The first step Julian took to reverse his fatigue and find quiet in a noisy world was to agree to go on a media diet. His overconsumption of media was leading to the downstream effects of fatigue, sleep problems, and mood changes, and we had to tackle the source of the problem.

When I see a stressed patient with limited mental bandwidth, prescribing a media diet is often my first intervention because of its ability to dramatically minimize stress and burnout. As we've seen, even if you don't suffer from media overconsumption like Julian, limiting the time you spend on your electronic devices has been shown to improve mental health and well-being.

The media diet is a three-part strategy—with time limits, geographical limits, and logistical limits—that I've prescribed to countless patients, and sometimes friends and family members, for many years with excellent results.

Time Limits: The first step for Julian was creating a time boundary for his media use. I prescribed only twenty minutes twice a day of media time for him. He set a timer on his phone and scrolled the headlines. When twenty minutes was up, he had to stop scrolling and put his phone someplace away from him.

Because constant scrolling had been such a large part of Julian's day, I knew this would be initially difficult for him. I suggested that he have an alternative activity that he loved to do close at hand. In Julian's case, he was a fan of a particular book series, so he decided he would read instead. Whenever he had the urge to pick up his phone to check the news, he planned to read at least a couple pages of his book. While he was still in my office for his first appointment, I also asked him to turn his phone screen to black and white or grayscale instead of multicolor. Today's news and media sites have made their content increasingly colorful, visual, flashy, and at times even shocking in the past ten years. It unmistakably hooks your attention. Making the screen black and white tones down some of that visual appeal. These were the plans Julian and I put into place for his first strategy. It seemed to work for him.

Geographical Limits: The second strategy was creating a physical boundary with Julian's phone by prescribing a few geographical limits. The first thing I asked him to do was to invest in a low-cost alarm clock rather than use his phone as an alarm so he could keep the phone off of his nightstand when he went to bed. He told me he would leave it plugged in on his desk on the other side of the room. I explained how this geographical boundary would put a circuit breaker on his now unconscious habit of grabbing his phone and scrolling through headlines before even getting up in the morning, which was setting the tone for the whole day. This would protect his mental bandwidth and give him a chance to start the day differently from how he had the past two years. Studies show that 62 percent of people check their phones within fifteen minutes of waking up, and about 50 percent check them in the middle of the night.[8] So keeping the phone off of his nightstand would also help his sleep.

During the day, especially while he was working, I recommended that Julian keep his phone more than an arm's length away and preferably out of sight altogether. This geographical boundary prevented him from automatically checking his phone.

Logistical Limits: The last step in Julian's media diet was creating a logistical boundary around his tech and media use, making his media use just a touch more inconvenient for him. He unsubscribed from all automated news alerts and push notifications, and he removed all dings, bells, and whistles alerting him of something new happening in the world of social media. This was another layer to remove the temptation of checking his phone.

When Julian came in for his follow-up appointment eight weeks later, he was well on course to mastering his media diet. He had begun to find his quiet in a noisy world.

"It was touch-and-go in the beginning," he told me. "Honestly, I didn't think I could do it. But I stuck to it and I can't begin to tell you what it's done for me."

"Good for you, Julian!" I cheered.

"I gradually cut down my phone time each day by thirty minutes. Then in four weeks, I was finally able to make it so that I was scrolling for only twenty minutes, twice a day," Julian told me.

"Did it get easier?"

"Well, I can tell you this, I read two whole books in my book series during the first ten days on this media diet," Julian said, laughing. "They're really good books!"

I asked Julian how he was sleeping at night.

"Putting my phone across the room on my desk might be the best thing I've ever done for myself," he said. "I usually read my book until I feel sleepy, which is now after a chapter or two. I still wake up quite a bit throughout the night, but I don't feel compelled to look at my phone."

I could visibly see the changes in his demeanor. He was more joyful, relaxed, and calm. It was clear that Julian had found his quiet and was relishing its discovery.

"I feel this huge sense of relief, like a weight's been lifted off of me," he said. "I feel like my old self again. I can finally breathe. I don't think I've taken a deep breath in two years. Does that make any sense?"

It made perfect sense, I reassured him. "Overconsuming tech causes your stress pathway to go into overdrive. It can make you irritable and hypervigilant. It looks like you've reset your stress response by all the great changes you've made."

Julian's experience lined up with the scientific research. In one study of 1,095 people, quitting Facebook for just one week improved life satisfaction and positive emotions, and these changes were most significant for heavy Facebook users, as Julian had been with other social media and news sources.[9]

The changes Julian made to his tech and media use also decreased his fatigue. He didn't need daily naps at work anymore, but his nighttime sleep still wasn't great. He woke up often throughout the night. Since he had slept with a TV on through the night for the previous six months, his sleep would need more time to change.

With his tech and media use in check, we agreed to keep building on the Rule of 2 for his next visit. He decided to prioritize his sleep and added a few more of my reset techniques (see below). When Julian followed up another eight weeks later, the media diet had become a new way of life. His sleep was much improved too. He reported very few nighttime awakenings and woke up feeling well rested.

"I always said I didn't have time to sleep more or to exercise," he told me. "But now that I'm off my phone, I have so much more time to do things that make me feel good. I haven't felt this optimistic in years!"

I saw Julian every two months to help him stay on track, and we watched together how his Personalized Stress Score (see Chapter 1) was gradually trending lower with each visit. Ultimately, Julian found his version of balance. He was able to consume media without it consuming him.

"I'm still a newsie. I always will be," Julian concluded. "But it's not messing with my life anymore. I finally feel like I'm the one who's in control!"

Julian was able to reset his stress and found a way to his best self. He had found some quiet in a noisy world. And as Julian proclaimed during one of his follow-up visits with me, "My barbecue friends are all hooked on this great book series now because I've been telling them all about it when we get together. I even leave my phone in my pocket the whole time I'm with them."

Our Primal Urge to Scroll

Julian's relentless attachment to his phone and excessive media use could easily be true for any of us. It's not your willpower that's the issue. Your biology is what strong-arms you into media overconsumption. When you're stressed, you are biologically wired to consume more media because having information can be a way of feeling safe. Even though the internet wasn't even invented until the 1990s, your urge to scroll is in your primal nature. As you now know, during periods of stress, your brain goes into survival mode and your lizard brain, the amygdala, takes over (see Chapter 2). Scrolling is the modern-day self-preservation equivalent of scanning your environment for danger in order to feel safe in a chaotic world.

In tribal cultures, a guard may have sat by the fire all night scanning for danger so the rest of the tribe could sleep. We are all that person now. And so we scan. All. Day. Long. In today's uncertain world, scrolling is the night watchman for our sense of safety.

Unfortunately, our primal urge to scroll ends up amplifying our stress response, which causes us to scroll some more, which then keeps the cycle going. It's a negative feedback loop on repeat. Clickbait works on the biology of stress. News consumption has a direct impact on our brain chemistry. You may have heard the term *doomscrolling*, which is obsessively scrolling social media or websites for bad news. Well, doomscrolling is powered by the same brain machinery as our fight-or-flight response and is activated during periods of stress.

This is the loop Julian found himself in, and the Second Reset got him out of it by recalibrating his primal urge to scroll, which in turn reset his brain's stress pathway.

Minimizing media use is not meant to disparage the critical importance of journalism or of wanting to stay informed citizens in this changing world. But at what cost? Certainly not at the cost of your mental health. I'm a big supporter of the media because health communication is my passion. Before I became a doctor, I wanted to be a journalist, and I've been lucky enough to pursue both of these interests. I've done hundreds of on-air appearances for NBC News, MSNBC, CNN Headline News, and CBS News especially to offer my professional advice as a doctor to the public during the pandemic. This behind-the-scenes experience has given me an insider's perspective of the process of making media for public consumption. Most media outlets are viable businesses, so the field aims to cover stories that are considered newsworthy, timely, and important to you as a media consumer. It's an attention economy, after all, and media companies know that keeping your attention matters. I firmly believe that journalism is a significant and valuable part of our culture. It gives voice to the many important issues in our world. However, you can love journalism and, in my case, partake in journalism, stay informed about the world, and still maintain your sanity.

There's a fine line between consuming and overconsuming media. If you don't know whether you're in a place where overconsuming media is creating unhealthy stress, I suggest you turn your attention to your canary symptoms. Do you have symptoms that might be attached to crossing the line into overconsumption? Do you think you may have a case of popcorn brain? Do you feel compelled to check your phone often? Do you feel like time is swallowed up when you meant to look at your phone for only a moment? Do you feel nervous or irritable if you don't have an internet connection at all times? Are you having more physical issues, like Julian's fatigue and irritability?

People have told me that, if they really take a look at their media usage, they've had multiple canaries calling attention to growing issues like: difficulty concentrating, poor memory, feeling on edge or, conversely, lethargic. Some have told me they feel anxious, moody, depleted, or have a sense of hopelessness. A few of my patients have no mental health manifestations when they consume too much media, but they say they have physical difficulties, like headaches, neck pain, shoulder pain, back pain, and eye strain. What song is your canary singing to get your attention about your media use? Take a minute or two to write down the canary symptoms that have been trying to alert you that you may be overconsuming media.

TECHNIQUE #4: Cure Your Popcorn Brain

Here's a plan you can follow to minimize your risk of developing, or to cure, popcorn brain:

1. Aim to spend no more than twenty minutes twice a day scrolling on your phone. At all other times, use your phone only for essential calls, texts, and emails. Set a timer and stay accountable. It's easy to lose track of time when you're in the digital space.

2. Opt out of push notifications and automatic pop-up features. Trust that if there's something you need to know about, you'll hear about it on your time.

3. While working, aim to keep your smartphone at least ten feet away from your workstation. At home, consider doing the same, especially when you're with your family members.

4. At bedtime, keep your phone off your nightstand. This will help prevent nighttime phone checks and also prevent you from reaching for your phone first thing in the morning. Tell family members or colleagues to call you if there's an emergency.

In the early days of your media diet, you'll have a strong urge to check your phone for no specific reason. Anticipate this need. Have a viable alternative quickly on hand: a notepad for doodling or a fidget toy. Pace quickly around the room or glance through a colorful magazine or book. Rewiring your brain and overcoming your primal urge to scroll is a major feat. Congratulate yourself each day for minimizing your risk of popcorn brain. In time, your stress will thank you because you'll be deciding who and what gets your attention, not a device in the palm of your hand.

The Cycle of Trauma

When a traumatic event inundates the news and is mentioned repeatedly on social media platforms, I often get calls or emails from patients who are having a bad reaction to the news cycle. For many people, it's not about how much news they're consuming, but rather what specific news content is in front of them all the time that can intensify their stress. This is especially true if you've had a traumatic life experience in the past. There's been such a clear pattern of this in my clinical experience that I can almost predict which of my patients will need support for their media-induced stress based on what's happening in the world.

Selma came into my office tearful and anxious. She had spent nearly every waking moment of the previous two weeks watching the public confirmation hearings for Brett Kavanaugh to become a judge on the US Supreme Court, when testimony was presented regarding allegations against him of sexual abuse. Selma was a forty-six-year-old devoted political activist with a long career. She had always cultivated a healthy relationship with media in her decades of work.

She explained, "News is just noise for me. To do the work I do, I need to know what's going on in the world, but I can't let it distract me. I've been doing this work through some really difficult times."

Selma stood up and paced my office a bit. "This confirmation hearing has blindsided me. I can't stop watching. I'm so anxious. I have palpitations. I couldn't go to work last week; I could barely get out of bed and function, because I'm sleeping only an hour or two every night. It honestly took everything I had to come in to see you today."

As it turns out, Selma had a history of sexual trauma in her twenties. Her media consumption of current events was an emotional trigger for past events, something she never expected to happen so many years later. Her self-preservation feedback loop was in overdrive.

Selma had been thriving right up to when she started paying attention to this kind of news. She was seeing a therapist every month, and a psychiatrist every three months. She had been on a small dose of medications for anxiety and depression for the previous ten years and was doing well.

Selma's media consumption of the SCOTUS hearings was triggering her trauma, something she had healed more than a decade before. "It all came flooding back," she told me. "It's like I'm going through it again. My body and brain remember like it was yesterday."

Because of the urgency and critical nature of the situation, Selma's mental health needed two immediate actions: seeing her therapist right away and discussing with her psychiatrist whether she needed to adjust her medications.

When I checked on Selma later that week, she had restarted trauma-informed therapy and was strongly considering increasing her medication dosage. For Selma, her stress cascade escalated quickly to the point of needing urgent medical attention from simply consuming, not overconsuming, the news. This highlights just how much of an impact media consumption can have on your brain and body. Selma's experience is one case that represents the importance of trigger warnings on sensitive media content.

More recently, I spoke to a woman whose eighty-eight-year-old grandmother was being triggered by images of war-torn Ukraine.[10] She had stopped wearing her doctor-prescribed mask for sleep apnea on account of seeing the ubiquitous images in the media from Ukraine and being reminded of memories of wearing a gas mask with her father during World War II. Her brain's stress pathway remembered the trauma that had occurred eight decades before!

You don't have to have a history of trauma to feel the intensity or effect of difficult or traumatic news. In our modern world, we're more hyperconnected than ever. You have the ability to obtain real-time, on-the-ground information about events happening thousands of miles away as you sit on your living room sofa. Your thinking brain, ruled by reason, recognizes the difference and registers the distance. But your amygdala, the emotional brain ruled by self-preservation, doesn't quite understand. It can process events as immediate threats and thereby activate your stress mechanism. For survivors of trauma, this is exponentially worse because of their prior lived experience. They are traumatized all over again.

I've witnessed this phenomenon so often in my clinical practice with patients that I spoke to a researcher who has studied the impact of media on the brain in large populations of people. Dr. Roxane Cohen Silver, a research psychologist at the University of California–Irvine, describes what's happening to us as a *cascade of collective traumas*. "It is extremely important for the informed [media] consumer to recognize that there may be psychological consequences to consuming all bad news all the time," Silver said. "With increased [media] exposure, we see increased distress, anxiety, hypervigilance, and other acute stress responses . . . The more [graphic] content people are seeing, the more distress they're exhibiting. The more distress they're feeling, the more they're drawn to the content. . . . It is a cycle."

Silver continued: "The one thing I'm not endorsing in any way is censorship. . . . The news is critical. . . . [But] people can make a conscious choice to monitor the amount of time they're spending engaged with the media . . . without being immersed in it over and over again."

Parenting Ourselves

The bad news isn't going anywhere. But we need a better way to manage this constant onslaught of information to protect our mental health and well-being, while still remaining informed and thoughtful citizens. It's not an easy balance to strike, but it can be done. It doesn't have to be complicated or fraught with angst. Just look at how easily and effortlessly we set screen limits for our children.

This generation of teenagers and young children are digital natives. They've grown up with video games, they use tablets and computers at school, and many have smartphones so that busy parents know their child can reach them.

Nicole, who had come to see me the year before, realized how much she was overconsuming media one evening when her family had gone to their favorite pizzeria. As they waited for their order to arrive, she looked up from her phone screen to see that her husband and twelve-year-old daughter were both scrolling on their phones, and her four-year-old son was tapping at a game on an iPad screen. The next week, when she visited my office, she said, "I realized my husband

and I were unintentionally role-modeling to our kids that looking at a device constantly is fine. I don't want them to develop popcorn brain like I had." Nicole had successfully incorporated a media diet in her life, and through it she understood the dangers of excessive online use and media consumption on the developing brains of her daughter and son.

The adult brain may not be developing in quite the same way as a child's, but it's still evolving and being shaped by external stimuli through the process of neuroplasticity (see Chapter 2). The studies on the impact of screens on adults and kids have similar outcomes: both adults and children experience worsened moods, more irritability, sleep disturbances, increased stress, and are more quickly angered. It's time we start parenting ourselves and rethinking what screen time is doing to our brains at any age.

Sleep as a Therapeutic Intervention

There's a club you really don't want to be a member of, but it's becoming more and more popular with each passing year. It's the club of sleep-deprived people, and its membership now includes one in three Americans. There are many reasons people lose sleep—chronic illness, the needs of caregiving, jet lag, night shifts, and emergencies—but almost half of Americans say stress is a culprit for their sleep deprivation.[11] If your sleep is being negatively affected by your unhealthy stress, you're not alone.

The good news is that gaining a deeper understanding of how stress impacts your sleep can help you overcome many of your sleep challenges. So you too can find quiet in a noisy world.

As you've seen with Julian and Selma, screen time is closely tied to sleep disruptions. The science shows a clear inverse relationship: the more media you consume, the more likely your sleep will be negatively affected. No matter the age group, from infants to older adults, studies confirm a negative association between screens and sleep.[12]

Our sleep is in direct competition with a screen from the moment we get up until we fall asleep. What is the first thing you do when you wake up? If you're like 87 percent of people, you're likely to be scrolling on your phone within five minutes of waking up, often before your eyes acclimate to the light of day.[13]

There may be a brief respite as you get ready for work, but chances are you spend your workday in front of another screen. And then, when you're finally ready to log off at the end of the workday, you may decompress with more screens. But as Julian and Selma found for themselves, scrolling isn't a benign and harmless act. It can activate the stress mechanism in your brain. Your reliance on any size of screen can have big implications for your ability to sleep well.

That was the case with Tanya, a graduate student who also worked part time and came to see me for her worsening sleep problems. With only six more months before graduation, Tanya's stress levels were high and she wasn't sleeping well, which was negatively affecting her academic performance.

She was exasperated: "I'm running on fumes. I'm seriously thinking of quitting grad school. I'm not sure how much more of this I can take."

Tanya walked me through her typical day. She was up at 7 a.m. after hitting the snooze button several times. She spent thirty minutes scrolling through her social media feeds on her phone and then rushed to her classes. She was in school until the early afternoon. After school, she worked at the local science museum until 7 p.m. She arrived home feeling depleted. "Like, every minute of my day is being accounted for by someone other than me," she declared.

She studied until 10 p.m. Then she would decompress from her long, stressful day in front of a screen—either her smartphone or the television—until 1 or 2 a.m. The next day, the cycle repeated itself.

"It hasn't always been this way," Tanya explained. "I used to be a great sleeper. I'm a Ph.D. student in physiology. I know all about the benefits of sleep. But now it seems like even if I'm exhausted, I just can't fall asleep before 1 a.m. and I'm tossing and turning all night long. It's like my brain doesn't want to shut off!"

"When we can have good days, only then can we have good nights," I explained.

Tanya hadn't allotted any time in her day to incrementally release her stress, so it became her constant bedfellow and made its presence known at night.

I used my tea kettle analogy from Chapter 1 to explain what was happening to her. "Your brain is like a tea kettle when it comes to how it responds to heightened periods of stress, like the final months of graduate school. You can't turn down the heat of the moment, right?"

"Not at this point," Tanya agreed. "I've got to finish my dissertation, and I have a number of exams coming up. Quitting my job isn't an option because I need it to pay my bills."

"So, let's view those as the external forces that you have no control over. They are on a timeline that's unchangeable," I said.

"The heat is turned on high in my life. I feel like I could burst," Tanya told me, starting to cry.

I continued: "Tea kettles don't explode because they have a steam release valve. Our work together is about my teaching you how to open the lever and blow off some therapeutic steam so the pent-up stress has someplace else to go besides your sleep."

Tanya wiped her eyes with equal parts relief and exhaustion. She was fully on board and ready to commit to the plan I had. Our shared goal was to fix her sleep so she could graduate on time with solid academic standing.

Tanya was experiencing three of the most common manifestations of sleep challenges all at once: difficulty falling asleep, difficulty staying asleep, and increased sleep fragmentation in the form of disrupted sleep. For Tanya, sleep loss was her canary.

For many people, disrupted sleep is one of the most common first signs of a maladaptive, unhealthy level of stress. Of the tens of thousands of stressed people I've communicated with over the years, sleep is by far the most common concern of anyone in the midst of a stress struggle.

You may not have trouble falling asleep like Tanya or have bedtime palpitations like I did, but chances are, if you're feeling the effects of maladaptive, unhealthy stress, it's likely that you're not sleeping as well as you once did.

The Sleep-Stress Cycle

Sleep and stress are so closely tied because they share a common culprit: *cortisol*. Known as the stress hormone, cortisol levels ebb and flow throughout the day to help you respond to whatever situation you're in. Just as stress can be healthy or unhealthy depending on the amount and frequency, so can cortisol. Cortisol isn't inherently bad; it's an important and necessary hormone for many daily functions. It's all about how much and how often it's being produced in your body.

When you're under stress, your adrenal glands (located above your kidneys) produce cortisol after they receive a signal from your brain's pituitary gland. Cortisol is released into your bloodstream and rushes in to turn on your fight-or-flight response. Cortisol has been hard at work throughout human history. When early humans were confronted by various dangers, such as a charging tiger, cortisol helped them escape. Cortisol cues the heart to pump blood faster to the large muscles of the body (like those in your legs) and mobilizes stored glucose to help the large muscles activate. It's a survival hormone, helping you to escape quickly or fight off the danger threatening you. For our early ancestors, once the danger was long gone, the acute stress was over and cortisol would return to normal, baseline levels.

The unique challenge of our modern world is that many of our stresses aren't acute, but chronic, so our stresses don't really pass, they simply accumulate. Cortisol, just like your amygdala, hasn't evolved with the times; it doesn't know that you're stressed about finances and not about a tiger chasing you. Chronic stress keeps your cortisol switched on in the background at a constant hum.

Cortisol's other big role in the body is to regulate your sleep cycle, so it's not hard to see how the constant threat of chronic stress can send your sleep cycle into a negative spin. Over time, your higher-than-usual cortisol levels start to impact your sleep, making it harder for you to fall asleep, stay asleep, and wake up feeling rested. This sleep-stress cycle continues night after night.[14]

If you're in the middle of your stress struggle, you know exactly what I mean—the all-too-familiar cycle of sleepless nights. You're stressed during the day and your body appropriately responds by increasing your cortisol production, which in turn affects your sleep, which then adds to your stress, which releases more cortisol.

The good news is that there are circuit breakers that have been proven to end this cycle. When you follow the Rule of 2, you can reset your sleep through managing your stress. It doesn't happen overnight, but it can happen with a little time, effort, and patience. With the Rule of 2, week by week, you can get your sleep back to what it used to be before your runaway, unhealthy stress took over.

The reason sleep is so important for your stressed brain is because it's *neuroprotective* for the brain, that is, sleep helps the brain stay healthy. Two researchers write in their article that the "fundamental purpose of sleep is to act like a garbage disposal for the brain. Essentially, sleeping acts as a garbage collector that comes during the night and removes the waste product [leftover proteins and metabolic by-products] left by the brain. This allows the brain to function normally the next day."[15]

Sleep helps you process difficult emotions and cope with the demands of life. Ironically, just when you're stressed and need the help of waste removal experts the most is when they go on strike. They take the night off, and your mental trash starts piling up.

We know much more about how sleep can impact your brain by studying what happens to your brain when you don't get enough of it. Sleep deprivation can slow your brain's capacity for cognition, concentration, memory, and attention.[16] It weakens your prefrontal cortex and makes your amygdala more reactive.[17] Brain scans of sleep-deprived people showed a 60 percent higher reactivity in the amygdala compared with well-rested brains when subjects were shown emotionally negative images.[18]

These brain findings might match up with what you experience with sleep deprivation: irritability, moodiness, and trouble regulating your emotions. The next time you say to someone, "I'm moody because I haven't been sleeping well," just know that it's your hyperreactive amygdala doing that.

Sleep deprivation doesn't negatively affect only your brain; it can also lead to negative consequences for your whole body, regardless of how old you are. Studies of teenagers have found links between sleep deprivation and higher blood pressure, abnormal cholesterol levels, and even insulin resistance, which is a precursor to diabetes.[19] Sleep-deprived adults have a 30 percent greater risk of developing chronic health conditions.[20]

How well you sleep, or how poorly you sleep, is also a predictor of your future mental health. Sleep-deprived teens and adults are more likely to suffer from current anxiety and depression but are also at greater risk for future depression.[21] In one analysis involving more than 170,000 adults, sleep disturbances doubled the risk of depression later in life.[22]

Although the science of sleep is clear and precise—your brain needs restorative sleep to function optimally—life can be messy and complicated. It's unrealistic to expect yourself to sleep soundly every single night, in spite of your best efforts. There will inevitably be nights when you don't get the sleep you need. You may be out late celebrating an event, traveling with jet lag, working on a crushing deadline, or tossing and turning because of a legitimate worry or concern. You may even set an early bedtime and have a poor night's sleep. What then? Science provides us with important guideposts, but we're ultimately mere mortals and not programmable robots. We're all doing the best we can. Don't let a few nights of poor sleep add to your stress and debilitate you. A few days, weeks, or frankly even a few months of inadequate sleep won't have lasting negative effects on your brain and body. These scientific warnings are for chronic sleep deprivation that lasts more than many months and maybe even years.

As you've seen with stress, your brain and body are designed to withstand acute, short-term stress very well. Common sleep disturbances often accompany short-term stress because of the sleep-stress cycle and cortisol. When you inevitably face stress and it affects your sleep (because it's as universal an experience as stress itself), be kind to yourself. Avoid berating yourself for not sleeping well, and let it go. Take the sleep disruptions as opportunities to practice self-compassion instead.

Focus on recovery on the days you're sleep-deprived. Consider frontloading your most important tasks to earlier in the day when you have more mental bandwidth to manage them. Set boundaries on your media consumption to give your brain a breather. Avoid over-exerting yourself physically and stay hydrated and well-nourished. If you must nap, ensure that it's a short nap and that you're not sleeping until late afternoon.[23] If you need caffeine to keep you going, avoid consuming it past 3 p.m. Both long naps and late-day caffeine consumption can interfere with your upcoming night's sleep.

On these low-energy, sleep-deprived days, give yourself some grace and try your best again tomorrow. Trust in your ability to find your way back to better sleep through the techniques in this chapter. With time, patience, and practice, you will reclaim your brain's ability for restorative sleep to find quiet in a noisy world.

"Tanya," I said, "I'm sharing the science of sleep with you to help you get ahead of your sleep deprivation before it has a lasting impact on you."

"Good! I'm not okay with my current sleep cycle messing with my future," Tanya told me. "I have lots of things I want to do after I graduate, so I need lots of energy."

Whatever hesitation Tanya felt at the start of our conversation, it dissipated when I shared the many reasons why focusing on her sleep was a key priority in her stress recovery now and in the future.

Tanya's goal was to start sleeping a full seven to nine hours every night, falling asleep more quickly and staying asleep throughout the night. It was a tall order, but I knew that by focusing on lowering her stress, we would also improve her sleep.

Bedtime Procrastination

The first step was to change Tanya's bedtime from 1 a.m. to earlier—preferably before midnight and closer to 10 p.m. Tanya had become anxious about her sleep and not sleeping well, so she kept pushing off her bedtime later into the night. "I know sleep is important, but I just can't seem to get myself to bed at a decent hour," she said with exasperation.

Tanya was engaging in a growing cultural phenomenon called *bedtime procrastination*. In one study of 308 patients, most of whom were women, bedtime procrastination had a strong correlation with those patients who were the most anxious.[24] They slept fewer hours per night and had more problems with sleep compared with patients who were less anxious. Surprisingly, the patients who engaged in bedtime procrastination acknowledged the importance of sleep but still couldn't manage to get to bed earlier.

This surprised the researchers. "We found that the majority of participants agreed that sleep is important," they noted. "On one hand, this is fantastic because it means we do not have to convince people why sleep is essential. On the other hand, it suggests sleep loss is more complicated than a matter of motivation."[25] (This is another case of what we've already seen with Wes: there's a gap between knowledge and action.)

These findings align with my own clinical experience. Nearly every patient I've helped with sleep deprivation wants to get to bed earlier, but for a myriad of reasons, they can't or won't.

"Of course you want more sleep," I reassured Tanya. "First, you need to break the cycle you're currently stuck in. We're going to find your circuit breakers together. You deserve a good night's rest."

Tanya relaxed her hunched shoulders and with tears in her eyes said, "You have no idea how much I need that rest."

Most of my patients with sleep problems can no longer ignore their canary, alerting them that they need to reset their stress. Sleep is the first area to focus on for their Rule of 2. They aren't looking for fancy, complicated theories of why they're not sleeping. They simply want a clear-cut, actionable plan to get the sleep they crave and need.

"Please, tell me what to do and I'll do it. I'm so tired of feeling tired," Tanya said with a big sigh, "I'm desperate for real rest." Tanya and I began with breaking the cycle of her bedtime procrastination, which was a major driver of her sleep deprivation. We focused on shifting her bedtime to earlier in the night. You have a twenty-four-hour cycle, an internal body clock that your body abides by, called your *circadian rhythm*. It's regulated by cortisol. Levels of cortisol ebb and flow throughout the day, but they are usually the lowest around midnight and the highest in the early morning hours between 6 and 8 a.m.

The first goal is to get in sync with your internal clock. That's where I started with Tanya. She already had her wake-up time of 7 a.m., but she was shortchanging her body clock by going to bed too late. By aiming for an earlier bedtime before midnight, she would reap the benefits of a sleep-wake cycle that was in sync with her body's natural circadian rhythm. Our wise ancestors who came up with the expression "one hour's sleep before midnight is worth two after" probably had a hunch about internal body clocks and circadian rhythms.

If your sleep-wake cycle resembles Tanya's, with a later-than-you-would-like bedtime, you're in good company. According to a colleague of mine in sleep medicine, it's one of the most common complaints he hears from his sleep-deprived patients. In fact, one conversation with him made me rethink my approach to patients when it comes to their sleep.

"I've asked hundreds of my patients these two questions and it's always the same response, every time," he said. "Ask your patients: 'What time do you go to bed now?' And follow it up with, 'What time would you ideally like to go to bed?' What you'll hear is a two-hour gap. Your patient may want to go to bed at 10 p.m., but they end up going to bed at midnight. When I probed further as to why this was, nearly every single person told me, 'I was using my phone/TV/laptop!' Screens are the chief enabler of bedtime procrastination," he said.

Can you relate? Is there a two-hour gap between your current bedtime and your ideal bedtime?

It makes perfect sense if there is. You probably don't have a lot of wiggle room when you wake up, because of work or family obligations or other appointments. But you do have a choice of wiggle room at bedtime. When you're stressed and burned out, you don't feel very powerful during the day. Every minute is accounted for, and often you're on someone else's schedule. But those glorious evening hours are yours and yours alone, to do whatever you want! That's a lot of power. So we stay up late as a form of "revenge" for our challenging days.

According to cognitive neuroscientist Lauren Whitehurst, this is a reaction to our hustle culture and inextricably tied to toxic resilience. "We value productivity so much that we pack our days," she says. "It's really a kind of commentary on [our lack of down time]."[26]

This resonated with Tanya, who had started our conversation telling me she didn't have enough time for herself, given the demands of school and work. "The only hours I have to myself are from 9 p.m. to midnight," she admitted. "I should be sleeping, but I need to decompress from my day before I can call it a day, you know?"

Of course, I knew. I've been guilty of staying up too late binge-streaming TV shows during my times of stress and burnout too. We're all human. In fact, my childhood best friends and I have a WhatsApp group with a steady supply of show recommendations we're enjoying. Our most common gripe is, "My sleep can't afford another show!"

But let's face it: sometimes it feels great to be a rebellious teenager again and stay up late even though you know it isn't good for you. When I'm captivated by a new show and staying up to binge-watch it, I give myself some grace. I hope you can find the compassion to do the same. I go to bed between 10 and 10:30 p.m. most nights, so a few nights with an 11:45 p.m. bedtime isn't a big deal. Sleep fluctuations are a part of life. A few late nights aren't going to throw off your sleep cycle. Your biology is resilient after all. The key is to get back on track with your ideal sleep routine as soon as possible, preferably right after you've finished bingeing that new series!

At first, when I suggested a 10 p.m. bedtime for Tanya, she was discouraged by my recommendation. It seemed like a big leap from her current 1 a.m. bedtime. She was desperate to find quiet in a noisy world but wasn't sure she could go through with it, even if her late nights contributed to her stress.

"You'll make this shift so gradually that it won't be jarring," I reassured her. "A few months from now, you'll realize you're in the groove of an earlier bedtime. It'll feel like it happened overnight, but there's nothing sudden about it. It's just your consistency and patience coming to fruition."

We needed to reset Tanya's sleep back to seven to nine hours a night, which is optimal for brain performance, instead of the five fitful hours of sleep in her current pattern. To get to an earlier bedtime, we looked at what Tanya was currently doing in the few hours leading up to bedtime. For her Rule of 2, we focused on two interventions: minimize her evening screen time and prioritize an earlier bedtime.

Tanya agreed to minimize her evening screen time by creating a relaxing bedtime routine instead. At my suggestion, she moved the TV out of her bedroom. Next, she set a timer for her bedtime screen time to one hour. Her eventual goal was to minimize all screen time two hours before bedtime. Two hours of no screen time before going to bed is optimal for restorative sleep, but for Tanya even one hour of screen-free time was a good step toward sleeping more soundly.

We needed to take into consideration what this change would feel like for Tanya. When you make even a small change in your established patterns or routines, you should anticipate feeling a resistance to that change, because your brain still wants to follow the neural pathway you already have in place. Tanya had been staying up until 1 a.m. for almost a year, so her neural pathway had grown strong with that repeated pattern. We discussed how she should anticipate resistance, and also the fact that nature doesn't like a vacuum, so she needed to replace her time on social media and TV with something that was relaxing.

Tanya told me she loved to stretch and do gentle yoga but had never figured out how to build it into her packed, everyday life. She had taken a few restorative yoga classes over the previous year and had learned some simple stretches that she could do at home. Since she had often complained to her friends that her shoulders and neck were tight after a day of studying hunched over her computer, a gentle stretching routine before bed seemed like the perfect opportunity to get her stretches in and help her body feel limber.

Tanya happily decided she would place a rolled-up yoga mat within easy reach in her bedroom to use as a substitute for screen time. Stretching would give her a moment of reset at the end of her overscheduled day to let go of her stress. The slow, deep breathing she'd use during her stretching sequence would also strengthen her mind-body connection (which is the basis of our Third Reset in the next chapter).

Instead of getting into bed with a tense body and overactive mind, Tanya would first stretch and then get into bed with relaxed muscles and a calm mind. This would have a ripple effect. It would help her fall asleep more quickly and stay asleep throughout the night.

Tanya loved the prospect of being fully relaxed in both body and mind. She left my office with a concrete plan in place, ready to find her quiet in a noisy world, and decided to implement the plan that very night. She even knew exactly which gentle stretching sequence she would do to launch her new routine.

The reason screens can be problematic for sleep is because they have two main mechanisms that interfere with your deep, restorative sleep: the first has to do with pure mechanics, and the second with psychology. First, screens of all types emit a frequency of light called *blue light*. Blue light activates the awake mechanism in your brain even if you're sleepy. You may have felt the very real effects of blue light on your brain's awake center if you've checked your phone at 3 a.m. and then, in spite of having just been in a deep sleep, your mind is alert even though your body is still exhausted. Blue light from the screen just sent a signal to your brain that it's time to wake up.

Blue light doesn't only affect your ability to stay asleep; it can also impact your ability to *fall* asleep. Tanya struggled with both. It's pretty easy to convince yourself that you're going to do a quick check of social media before bed and then find yourself an hour or two later finally signing off. Suddenly, your 10 p.m. bedtime has become midnight or much later as your brain tries to decipher whether it's time to sleep or to stay awake. This isn't a failing of your brain. In fact, your brain is working exactly as it should be when exposed to blue light. Remember, the primary goal of media of any kind is to keep you engaged as a viewer, and the blue light from your electronic device is doing exactly that—keeping your brain focused on the external content in front of you, rather than the internal need for sleep within you.

Sometimes, putting your phone away for the night might not be an option. You may have elderly parents, teenagers, or young adult kids who you want to be sure can reach you at any time. I understand. As a doctor, I've often been in a position where I've had to check my messages and emails during late hours. But you can still be available on your device without fully activating the wake-up daytime biology in your brain. Most phones have a way to set your phone to bedtime or night mode or to set a night light or blue light filter. I have my own phone switch to this option between 8 p.m. and 7 a.m. This way, at 8 p.m. every evening, my phone filters out the blue light and replaces the display with warmer orange tones. Then, in the morning it automatically returns to the default display of blue light. Another method to consider is using glasses with lenses that block blue light. Neither of these options is 100 percent effective at filtering all blue light, but they are workable alternatives when staying off your phone overnight isn't an option for you.

The second reason why bedtime screen time interferes with sleep is less about biology and more about psychology.[27] At the end of her day, Tanya felt depleted, worn out, and stressed. When she finally had a moment to herself, what was the easiest thing to do with the least effort to decompress from the day's events? Numb out in front of her screens, of course! The unfortunate consequence of decompressing this way is that it can lead to that delayed bedtime that Tanya was trying to overcome. Many factors influence revenge bedtime procrastination, such as individual coping skills, the flexibility in your job, and how much of your day you feel you can control.[28] Parents with young children at home may savor those kid-free hours after the kids are asleep and extend their own bedtimes well past the midnight hour. But even with all of these individual moving parts, the biggest driver in your brain for revenge bedtime procrastination is your inescapable burnout and stress.[29] Sleep is the very thing your brain needs when facing burnout and stress because sleep helps the brain process difficult emotions. It's also important for learning, cognition, memory, attention, and nearly every function in the human body. Sleep truly impacts every cell, muscle, and organ system in the body, including the brain. The benefits of restorative sleep for burnout and stress cannot be overemphasized, yet sleep is often the first thing to be hurt by burnout and stress.

Tanya's second Rule of 2 was to prioritize an early bedtime to increase her sleep duration. As noted, the ideal amount of sleep for optimal brain and body function is seven to nine hours per night. "Protecting your sleep now is something your future self will thank you for," I told Tanya.

In addition to the benefits of sleep for her brain, we also discussed how enough sleep could help Tanya's heart. She was young and her heart was currently in great shape, but she also had a family history of heart disease. Both of her grandfathers, three uncles, and her aunt had suffered from heart problems. I shared the results of a recent study with her that encouraged her further to make the big change to an earlier bedtime of 10 p.m. We agreed on aiming for a bedtime between 10 and 11 p.m., which, according to some new compelling research, may be the "golden hour" for sleep.

In the study I shared with Tanya of almost ninety thousand people, researchers found that bedtimes between 10 and 11 p.m. were linked to better heart health, while bedtimes after midnight were linked to a 25 percent higher likelihood of heart problems.[30] According to lead researcher David Plans, "the results suggest that early or late bedtimes may be more likely to disrupt the body clock, with adverse consequences for cardiovascular health."[31]

Tanya was ready to reset her body clock because she now understood how critical sleep was to her being able to function at a high level for school and work. Tanya's new bedtime of 10 p.m. was going to be a big change, but I promised we'd get there taking small steps.

Tanya was able to slowly shift her bedtime from 1 a.m. to 10 p.m. over three months by following a sleep schedule that shifted her bedtime by thirty minutes every two weeks so her body and brain could gradually acclimate. Weeks 1 and 2, Tanya aimed for a 12:30 a.m. bedtime. For weeks 3 and 4, she shifted to a midnight bedtime. Every two weeks she subtracted another half hour from her bedtime procrastination and added it to her healthy amount of sleep. By week 11, Tanya was comfortably in bed at 10 p.m.

In addition to the above interventions, I also reiterated the basics of "sleep hygiene" that most doctors share with their patients. Many of these Tanya was already doing, but they served as good reminders:

- Create a relaxing bedtime routine.
- Keep your bedroom dark and cool.
- Use your bed for sleep and sex only, not for eating, work, or other activities.
- If possible, remove the TV from your bedroom.
- Avoid caffeine after 3 p.m., and minimize alcohol and nicotine use.
- Aim to do physical activity every day, but preferably no strenuous aerobic exercise in the evening.
- If you must nap, keep naps short and nap earlier in the day so napping doesn't interfere with nighttime sleep.
- If your sleep problems continue, consider seeing a sleep specialist.

When Tanya came to see me for a follow-up, her Personalized Stress Score had dropped significantly, and she felt less stress. She attributed this to her new sleep schedule. "I actually feel as proud of myself for improving my sleep habits as I do for my grade point average," Tanya told me. "Which has also increased," she added with a smile.

"Many of my patients say, 'There aren't enough hours in the day to do it all,'" I responded. "But the truth is, when you give your brain the sleep it needs, your focus improves and you can get more done in a shorter amount of time."

Tanya continued with early bedtimes, with the occasional late night during exam week or for social events. Since Tanya's better sleep had become a habit, she could be back on track with her sleep after the blip, which is a normal and expected part of having a full life.

Through only two incremental changes using the Rule of 2, Tanya made huge strides in her sleep over three months and achieved her goals. She graduated on time, with excellent academic standing. She's now working full time at a demanding, high-stress job but continues to minimize her screen time and protect her sleep like the vital and precious resource it is.

TECHNIQUE #5: Get the Sleep You Deserve

1. Aim for a 10 p.m. bedtime. If your current bedtime is after midnight, slowly set your bedtime thirty minutes earlier every two weeks until you reach your ideal bedtime.

2. Set a bedtime alarm approximately one hour before your intended bedtime to encourage you to start transitioning into sleep mode.

3. Create a relaxing bedtime routine. Reading a book before bed can encourage restful breathing, improve stress, and minimize psychological distress. You might also consider listening to

relaxing music or practicing some gentle yoga stretches, both of which prime the brain for rest, signaling your sleep mechanism to kick in.

4. Aim to minimize evening screen time, particularly two hours before bedtime, to prevent the awake mechanism in your brain from being artificially activated by the blue light emitted by screens of all kinds.

5. Keep your phone off your nightstand and use a separate, low-cost alarm clock instead. This will help you avoid checking your phone in the middle of the night and prevent you from scrolling the moment you're awake in the morning.

6. Remove your TV from your bedroom if possible. If you do watch TV in the bedroom, limit the amount of time you watch it.

7. Reap the many mental health and physical health benefits of your new and improved sleep schedule. Your stress and burnout will begin trending in a new direction!

Your Sleep-Deprived Brain

Like Tanya, my patients who have suffered from sleep deprivation are often fraught with worry. When you're not sleeping well, it's normal to fixate on your sleep disturbances. Bedtime becomes a high-stress event with lots of foreshadowing mixed with doom and gloom:

What if I can't fall asleep again tonight?

What if I keep waking up during the night?

What if I wake up exhausted again?

What if I can't sleep through the night ever again?

If you're sleep-deprived, these common what-ifs, along with so many others, can keep you anxious and awake when you are trying to sleep. This is a normal psychological reaction called *anticipatory anxiety*. It's the dread and angst you feel when you're thinking about something that's coming up. You can have anticipatory anxiety about anything, because anxiety is a future-focused emotion. It's fueled by "what-ifs." But when you're not sleeping well, your lack of sleep can biologically also make you more anxious.[32]

It's an experience researchers call *overanxious and underslept*.[33] In one study of healthy volunteers, anxiety levels in sleep-deprived people increased by 30 percent after one night of no sleep, and 50 percent of people met the criteria for an anxiety disorder.[34] As it turns out, the sleep-deprived brain and the anxious brain have a lot in common. In the study, brain scans of healthy, sleep-deprived people revealed something new and interesting: the same brain regions that are overactive in anxiety, like the amygdala, are overactive in sleep deprivation. Conversely, the same brain areas that are underactive in anxiety, like the prefrontal cortex, are underactive in sleep deprivation.

"Sleep loss triggers the same brain mechanisms that make us sensitive to anxiety," said researcher Eti Ben Simon. "When we're well-rested, regions that help us regulate emotions are the ones that help keep us calm. Those regions are very sensitive to sleep loss. Once we're losing sleep, these regions are going offline. We're not able to trigger those processes of emotion regulation."[35]

Remember, that ancient cave dweller lizard brain, your amygdala, is a key driver in your stress pathway, and your prefrontal cortex helps to quell an overactive amygdala. With these new brain scan findings, scientists discovered the fascinating role of deep, therapeutic sleep: it's an anxiety inhibitor that helps your brain reset from stress.[36]

New information is being discovered every day about how our biology affects our sleep. So it's not you. It's your biology. Give yourself some grace.

I wish I had taken my own advice when I was struggling with sleep as a new mom. In the months following the birth of my child, I was fraught with worry about sleep deprivation. The more I worried about the upcoming night's sleep, the more stressed I became, the worse I would feel, and the poorer I would sleep.

One conversation with a colleague, a sleep medicine physician who had given birth a few years earlier, set me straight. I confessed to her over lunch that I wasn't sleeping well. I surprisingly felt a lot of shame around my inability to sleep. I preached the benefits of sound sleep to patients, so how was I not able to sleep well myself in spite of following my own sleep prescription?

I braced myself for her judgmental reaction as a sleep medicine expert.

She laughed and hugged me instead. "I didn't sleep for a year after my baby was born!" she said. "Do the best you can and don't sweat it. You'll get a good night's rest eventually."

I felt a great sense of relief. Her words gave me the permission I needed to give myself the same grace I give my patients. I let go of my expectation of a perfect night of sleep.

It turns out, she was right. Data from a new study show that parents can be sleep deprived for up to six years after the birth of their child.[37]

When I took the pressure off myself to sleep well, I started to sleep better. The approach I used on myself was the same I use with my patients. I stopped fixating on the quality of my nights and started to focus on the quality of my days. I started exercising again after work and meditating during my lunch breaks. When I started to have better days, I had better nights. I got better at sleeping through the back door.

This back door approach has worked for so many of my patients.

If you're anxious and feeling like you're on a relentless loop of worrying about sleep, or suffering from sleep deprivation, I invite you to follow the sleep prescription in Technique #5 above with a healthy amount of self-compassion. I also encourage you to try the other strategies in this book that have nothing specific to do with sleep, like exercise or the 4-7-8 breathing technique (see Chapter 5), because they may help to offset your stress, which in turn could reset your sleep.

Hyperconnected Is Disconnected

Through social media, you may know quite a bit about what's going on in the lives of your friends, extended family, and classmates from the past, but that digital catchup actually has its share of negative consequences. If the data are any indication, you're probably spending more hours a day on your phone and fewer hours sleeping, but you're probably also spending more hours alone than ever before.

According to economist Bryce Ward, until a decade ago, Americans spent the same amount of time with friends as people did in the 1960s.[38] Then in 2014, there was a noticeable change, as Americans started spending more and more time alone. Why was 2014 the year that our social habits changed? That year was a tipping point in smartphone use—the first year that the majority of Americans, more than 50 percent, started using smartphones.[39] Since 2014, we've seen a stepwise, incremental rise in how many Americans use smartphones. These two trends aren't precise and causally related: you're not spending more time alone just because you're using your phone more. But studies have shown a correlation between the two.[40] And when we spend more time alone, we're more likely to experience low moods, trouble sleeping, and worsening stress.

Clearly, according to such studies, we're becoming hyperconnected when it comes to technology and increasingly disconnected when it comes to one another. Scientists can't pinpoint what this means for our long-term mental health and stress, but my hunch is that it's making our loneliness epidemic worse.

Over the past decade, we've seen a rise in loneliness around the world. Globally, at least 330 million adults go two weeks before speaking to a friend or family member.[41] In the United States, loneliness has become such a pressing concern that the Surgeon General issued an advisory, calling loneliness a public health crisis.[42] Recent estimates suggest that one in two US adults reports feeling lonely, with Gen Z reporting even higher rates of loneliness—a whopping 78 percent![43]

A complex relationship exists between loneliness and stress, with studies showing that loneliness can worsen your stress.[44] There are also other health implications of loneliness. It's been found to increase your risk of developing heart disease by 29 percent and your risk of having a stroke by 32 percent. It holds the same risk of death as smoking fifteen cigarettes per day.[45] Loneliness can also shorten your lifespan. One study found that loneliness could increase your risk of premature death from every cause. Lead researcher Kassandra Alcaraz confirmed, "The magnitude of risk presented by social isolation is very similar . . . to that of obesity, smoking, . . . and physical inactivity."[46] Given these findings, we need an urgent fix for loneliness!

I've witnessed this play out so often in my clinical practice. Loneliness has been pervasive among many of my stressed patients, and addressing it, either through prevention or recovery efforts, has been a major part of my clinical work. I ask every patient this question about their social support: "Do you feel like you have friends you can trust and lean on during difficult times?" Many of my patients say no. When I ask them to describe their closest friend, some have told me, "I don't have a best friend. If I did, it would be you, Dr. Nerurkar."

This answer reflects our current loneliness epidemic. We long for close associations. Knowing someone cares about what's going on in your life can be a great comfort. I've often wondered how much social isolation contributes to the statistic that 60 percent to 80 percent of doctor visits have a stress-related component. If patients had more social support and a greater sense of belonging, would doctors see so many stress-related visits? I'm not sure, but I don't think so.

Social support is so critical to your stress management that I include it as a main section in your Lifestyle Snapshot ("Your Sense of Community," see Chapter 2). You may have different social needs and thresholds—some of us are introverts while others are extroverts—but irrespective of our personality traits, feeling a sense of community and connection with others can help us thrive. The quality of your human relationships is the single greatest predictor of your happiness across your lifespan according to the Harvard Study of Adult Development, the longest-running study on happiness, spanning more than eighty years.[47] Social support is also reciprocal. As important as it is to have social support, being a source of social support for others can also improve your health.[48]

It's easy to feel isolated or prefer to be alone when you're stressed. But connecting with others from time to time can help decrease your stress, even if you're an introvert. There are many ways to cultivate meaningful connections. Consider incorporating simple moments of connection throughout your week. Chat with a neighbor, phone a friend to check in, join a local art class or another group, invite a colleague for a lunchtime break, or spend an afternoon at a flea market with a friend or family member.

If life feels too busy to be social, schedule social connections into your week. Each week, make at least one plan to connect with someone you enjoy during that week. Whatever you choose, find something that can lead to conversation and connection. Find a simple way to initiate a connection with someone else. You don't have to become a social butterfly, but your stress and burnout will benefit from a little more human connection in your life. Humans are wired for social connection, so cultivating our sense of belonging can help us thrive mentally and physically.

Let go of the myth that you have to be constantly productive or have a specific purpose for connecting with others and having some fun. That's a remnant of hustle culture. Science journalist Catherine Price says, "We typically think of fun as something that we can only have or experience when things are already going well. Actually, fun can boost our resilience and our spirits in a way that makes it easier for us to cope with whatever life may throw our way."[49]

Selma, my patient who was retraumatized by watching the Supreme Court confirmation of Brett Kavanaugh, spent countless hours as a political activist, which is almost always an intense effort. The people she spent the most time with were all on a serious and fierce mission to create political change. The next time she visited my office, Selma had applied the media diet to her life and was seeing improvements in her stress and sleeping. I suggested she add another item to her Rule of 2—a strategy to expand her social support to include enjoyment.

"What do you do to relax and enjoy yourself?" I asked Selma.

"Well, let's see . . . the last thing I did for fun was to go to a Fourth of July concert," Selma told me. "I took some disadvantaged youths from a social service agency, so I was chaperoning."

"The Fourth of July was six months ago, Selma. And chaperoning doesn't sound all that relaxing to me," I remarked gently, understanding now that Selma didn't allow time for her own joy.

"It wasn't very relaxing," Selma admitted. "The older kids kept sneaking off to smoke cigarettes."

We both laughed a bit. But I knew I had to take a different approach.

"Okay, let's shift to a different time in your life. Was there anything that made you happy when you were a teenager?" I asked.

"Oh, yes! I was on a trophy-winning soccer team in high school," Selma told me, grinning. "We were good! My new next-door neighbor, Alice, is getting an adult women's team together. She asked me if I wanted to join."

"Why not? You might love it again."

"I'm thirty years older now! What if I suck at soccer?" Selma said with a suppressed giggle.

"I don't think Alice would have asked you if she was worried about that," I told her.

"Well, maybe I'll call her," Selma said with some apprehension.

"Why not today?"

Selma stood up with determination, "Yes. Today. You know, my whole adult life I thought I had to put all my energy into political causes, be serious, and not waste time with hobbies or things that 'don't matter.'"

"Even when all of your energy is focused on a good cause, it can still become a source of unhealthy stress and burnout," I said. "We all need to reset by doing some form of self-care, and sometimes that includes doing things with other people just purely for fun."

Two months later, I saw Selma in my office again. She showed me a photo of her, Alice, and two other women in matching soccer jerseys. Then she thanked me for helping her remember how to enjoy herself again.

"My soccer league is fun," Selma told me, "but the best part is that Alice and I carpool to the games every week and we stop at a place that makes smoothies on the way home and try different flavors. We talk about life. And we laugh a lot. It's simple, but I feel so much happier."

"So, I take it you didn't suck at soccer?" I asked her, laughing.

"I don't. In fact, I feel like my body is thanking me for the opportunity to kick that soccer ball down the field with everything I've got," Selma said. "Doing this physical exercise has made me feel stronger emotionally, too. And I've met some cool, like-minded women who play each week in the league. We're planning a girls' trip to LA to see their women's soccer team!"

Selma's descriptions of soccer had me thinking about how every soccer match is an opportunity that's ripe with the possibility of a weekly reset. Through small steps, two at a time, Selma learned to protect her mental bandwidth using the techniques in the Second Reset. She found her quiet in a noisy world. She incorporated the elements of the media diet to overcome her primal urge to scroll, and reclaimed her brain and body's need for rest and healing in the process. Since she no longer felt depleted, she was able to use her mental bandwidth to build meaningful connections through her soccer league. By focusing on disconnecting online, Selma found connection and a sense of belonging, and fun, offline.

Selma had made a big leap forward and was now experiencing the benefits of the Third Reset—how to sync her brain and her body to keep her unhealthy stress in check—which we'll explore next!

5

The Third Reset: Sync Your Brain and Your Body

Your stress and burnout may feel bleak and permanent, but the good news is that both are fully reversible. You can reverse the negative impact of chronic stress on your brain and body by understanding the Third Reset: how to sync your brain and your body through the mind-body connection, which is the scientific premise that so much of this book is based on.

Of course, we all know that our brains are housed within our bodies, but we often forget how strongly one affects the other. You experience the mind-body connection for yourself almost constantly. Feeling your heart race before a big meeting, experiencing butterflies when you first fall in love, blushing during an embarrassing moment, and even having a gut reaction that something is right or wrong for you—these are all stand-out examples of your mind-body connection at work. Paradoxically, the mind-body connection, which is the foundation of this Third Reset, is often considered inconsequential to our levels of stress and our overall health.

The mind-body connection isn't a woo-woo concept; it's the

research-backed understanding that your brain and your body are in constant communication and inextricably linked. The HPA axis—the connection between your hypothalamus, pituitary gland, and adrenal glands (see Chapter 2)—is a concrete example of the mind-body connection, because it quite literally connects parts of your brain with your body. One key tenet of the mind-body connection is that what's good for your body is good for your brain and vice versa. When you do better, you feel better. And it's all in the doing.

Whether you're aware of the exchange or not, your brain is continuously sending signals to your body, and your body is responding accordingly. Just like gravity, the mind-body connection is a law of nature—it runs in the background, making your life possible in the foreground.

Plug in to the Mind-Body Connection

Wouldn't it be great if you could influence this cross talk to rewire your brain to beat your stress and burnout in the process? It turns out, you can. Even though the mind-body connection is an effortless natural phenomenon, plugging in to it with intention may feel unnatural at first. This is why it's part of our Third Reset: you can learn how to sync your brain and your body to strengthen your mind-body connection and overcome your unhealthy stress.

With the exception of elite athletes, most of us spend much more time living in our heads than in our bodies. Your body and brain send signals to each other all day long, but you seldom stop to recognize the messages. Once you perceive the way the mind-body connection works, however, and you see how it happens, you won't be able to unsee it—which is a good thing since there are a multitude of ways you can harness that connection to reset your brain and body for less stress and more resilience.

Let's revisit my own stress struggle as a doctor in training that I shared in Chapter 1. While working long days and nights as a medical resident, my only objective was to keep going. I told myself, *Keep doing it all and being it all. You're going to make it through medical training, and you'll succeed.* But I was regularly experiencing bedtime heart palpitations, which left me sleep-deprived and depleted. I wondered whether I had a cardiac issue, but I continued to push myself to work long, tedious hours. I was so far down the hole of stress and burnout that I didn't pay attention to my canary symptoms, which were telling me to stop and reset. I pressed on, despite the symptoms, because I thought discomfort was a normal part of medical training. My brain and body were talking to each other, but I just worked harder in an effort to silence their conversation. My brain and my body might as well have been screaming into a void.

I had never heard about the mind-body connection before. It wasn't a part of my training curriculum nor talked about much in conventional medicine during the early 2000s. Learning about this important connection was my last resort. Having the requisite medical tests and being told everything was "normal" didn't end those stampeding wild horses. So like many of my patients, I started doing my own research. As a doctor in training, I had access to an armamentarium of research studies and didn't need to use Dr. Google, as many of my patients do. I read about the scientific underpinnings of the mind-body connection and learned about the Mindfulness for Healthcare Providers class I mentioned in Chapter 1.

When I first saw the ad for the class, I thought, "Why not? It's on my way home from work. It's once a week for eight weeks. It's not that expensive. If I don't like it, I can bail after the first week."

But after that first class, not only couldn't I wait to attend the next one, but it felt like an eye-opening experience that altered the trajectory of my medical career.

The instructor, Dr. Michael Baime, seemed to understand that most of us fellow physicians in the class would require a simple first step for revealing and resetting the mind-body connection. We needed something that we could do, even in the middle of our hectic and overscheduled days, without having to set aside a specific period of time or step away from our work or home lives to do it. He taught us a technique that I used the very next day and that I've been using every single day since.

There's no better way to understand the mind-body connection in action than the Stop–Breathe–Be technique. It takes only a few seconds to learn and can help anyone begin to regulate and reset their mind-body connection in the moment for less stress and more resilience.

TECHNIQUE #6: Stop–Breathe–Be

The big-picture goal is to use this technique when doing a task that initiates events that might spark stress in your life. Choose a small, mindless, and repetitive task you do every day. It's ideal to pick something that can be the initiator of a cascade of events such as making coffee, cleaning your kitchen countertop, getting into your car, checking email, logging in to a virtual work meeting, or packing up your briefcase or backpack for the day ahead. The more mindless and repetitive the action, the better the result. My personal favorite is picking up my phone to check work emails.

As you're about to start the task, say to yourself in your mind or aloud the word *STOP.* Intentionally, bring your body to a full and complete stop. Pause and be as motionless as possible and become aware of your stillness in that moment.

Then say to yourself, *BREATHE.* Of course, you've been breathing all along, but take a few seconds to become fully aware of your breathing as you take one deep breath in and then let it all the way out. Try to relax your body as you take a deep breath.

Finally, say the word *BE*. Take the moment to ground yourself and be present. Bring your attention to that moment in time and relish the temporary pause. Simply become aware of yourself before you move on to the task you're about to do.

The Stop–Breathe–Be technique only takes about five seconds of pause, presence, and stillness, yet it can be an amazingly effective way to reset your stress using the mind-body connection. It's like a personal check-in from you to you.

When I first started using the Stop–Breathe–Be technique, I was working in a busy medical clinic, and the task I chose as my check-in with myself was the moment right before I knocked on the exam room door before entering to see a patient. When I reviewed my daily packed schedule of patients, it was easy to initially feel overwhelmed, and with time, experience the burnout so many doctors say they have. The Stop–Breathe–Be technique transformed my relationship to my work, my capacity to stay present with each patient, and my stress. For the first time, it unlocked my ability to activate my mind-body connection.

The start of each patient visit became a fresh, new opportunity for me to practice plugging in to my own mind-body connection. Those five seconds, repeated throughout the day, reset my mental bandwidth and allowed me to stay present in the moment, which completely changed the flow of my day. I was still just as busy with patient care, but I didn't feel as frenetic moving from one patient room to another.

When I started to practice Stop–Breathe–Be, I would stand at the doorway of my patient's room and, before knocking, would say to myself under my breath: "*Stop, Breathe, Be*" and follow the prompts as I've described. Over time, it became a habit, so I didn't need the verbal cues for myself.

This technique, done repeatedly throughout my long workday, reset the entire tenor of my workday and it had ripple effects throughout my whole life. Once I got the hang of Stop–Breathe–Be at work, I added some home tasks to the mix. I practiced it when I opened the blinds each morning, with my first cup of morning tea, as I cleaned my kitchen counter after cooking, and while I washed the dishes. I carried the five seconds of Stop–Breathe–Be into every corner of my mundane, everyday activities.

The funny thing about the mind-body connection is that it sounds like a glamorous concept, but actually, achieving a strong mind-body connection is pretty unglamorous. Such mundane repetitive tasks have so much power to transform our lives! And that's precisely why I get so excited about the stress-reduction techniques in this book. These tools are accessible to everyone at any time. You don't need a fancy spa, a mountaintop retreat, or even a high-tech gadget with artificial intelligence capabilities. You can reset your brain and body for less stress and more resilience using your newly learned techniques, such as Stop–Breathe–Be, which you can do using a pile of dirty laundry or dishes in front of you.

I advised Gabrielle, a thirty-three-year-old special needs teacher, to try Stop–Breathe–Be at work. She was telling me that the intense energy of her group of seven- and eight-year-olds, all on the autism spectrum, would often make her feel overwhelmed. She was starting to feel burned out by the constant demands of her job. I asked her to practice Stop–Breathe–Be every time she physically turned toward the blackboard.

Later, she said, "Having those five seconds throughout the day to connect back to myself has made all the difference. I use it at least a few dozen times a day. I'm going to teach it to the kids next."

It may only be a short five seconds, but the Stop–Breathe–Be technique packs a long-lasting punch. It activates your mind-body connection because it trains your brain to notice your body and its physical sensations, along with your thoughts and emotions, in that precise moment, rather than mindlessly barreling forward like we all usually do. In that moment, it helps to regulate your stress response by asking you to take a brief inventory, and through your breath, it helps you regulate your nervous system away from stress. A complex biological phenomenon is at play during Stop–Breathe–Be.

Did you know that your breath is the only physiological bodily process that is under both voluntary and involuntary control? You're able to voluntarily control your breathing (like taking a deep breath), but when you don't pay attention to your breathing, your body takes over for you involuntarily. How cool is that? No other bodily function can do that—not your heart beating, your gut digesting, or your brain thinking. This marvel of your human body is why your breath is the gateway to tapping into your mind-body connection.

Research also shows that your breathing patterns can influence your emotions.[1] For many years, scientists have known this process happens through the stress hormone cortisol, along with the vagus nerve, which has many roles in your body, including managing your breathing, digestion, and even your ability to relax.

While scientists long ago had identified cortisol and the vagus nerve as key players in how your breath is linked to your emotions, they weren't able to pinpoint exactly what was happening in the brain. Recently, a new study changed that. A group of scientists at Stanford University were able to pinpoint a small cluster of brain cells, which they called the *pacemaker for breathing*, that is responsible for linking your breath to your emotional state.[2] It's an important discovery that has been able to give us a much clearer cellular picture of what's happening in your brain when you breathe deeply, and how your breathing can help you manage your unhealthy stress. Your brain's pacemaker for breathing is the home of your mind-body connection, and your breath is a gateway to tap into it.

The Stop–Breathe–Be technique is incredibly effective at activating your mind-body connection incrementally over time, but you also need a few more tools at your disposal when you're faced with highly charged and intensely stressful moments.

TECHNIQUE #7: Breathe Easy

Here are a trio of techniques—diaphragmatic breathing, 4-7-8 breathing, and heart-centered breathing—that you can use as a stress prescription no matter where you are. I've practiced each of these in a business meeting, while driving, making dinner, hurrying for an appointment, and even while watching a movie with other people. No one will even notice you doing them.

Diaphragmatic Breathing

The most effective breathing technique to immediately put the brakes on your stress response *in the moment* during chaotic, heavy, or overwhelming situations is called *diaphragmatic breathing*—which is just a fancy name for deep belly breathing. When you're stressed, your breath becomes quick and shallow and stays only in the chest. When you're calm, your breathing is slower and deeper and comes from the belly. Babies are excellent diaphragmatic breathers, but somewhere in our development into adulthood, that changes. But you can learn to temporarily, voluntarily control the shallow, quick breathing that happens when you're anxious or stressed to short-circuit your stress response by switching to diaphragmatic breathing.[3]

Here's how you can practice diaphragmatic breathing:

1. Place your hands on your belly as you're learning this technique to help guide you.

2. Breathe in through your nose and let your belly rise while breathing in. Then exhale through either your nose or your mouth and let your belly fall as you breathe out.

You'll notice that as you practice diaphragmatic breathing, you start to take slower, deeper breaths from your belly area rather than from your chest. Because slower, deeper breathing can't coexist with anxious, shallow, and quick breathing, when you actively practice diaphragmatic breathing during stressful or overwhelming moments, you're dialing down your stress at the exact moment you need it.

Ryan, my patient from Chapter 3 who was a music industry executive, called me from London one afternoon. He was in a panic. "I've been sleeping much better, doing my daily prescribed walk and playing my guitar almost every day. It's been great," Ryan told me. "But I still have this anxiety in meetings and talking to other people. I'm supposed to connect in person with radio producers before the show today, but I'm dreading it. I've been kicking myself all day for being weak. I never used to be this way."

Over the phone, I could hear Ryan barely able to catch his breath.

"Okay, Ryan," I calmly said, "let's slow down your runaway stress right now. I'm going to teach you how you can overcome your fight-or-flight response and let your rest-and-digest response take over."

"How are you going to do that?"

"We're going to use your biology to work for you rather than against you so you can feel calm going into today's meetings. You're beating yourself up because your biology is actually trying to protect you."

Over the phone, Ryan and I practiced diaphragmatic breathing together. I asked him to place his hands on his belly, and to make sure his breath was traveling down from his chest into his belly such that he could feel his belly rise and fall with his breathing. In his acutely intense moment of stress, Ryan was learning how to activate his parasympathetic nervous system.

The *parasympathetic nervous system* leads to your "rest-and-digest" response. It works in direct opposition to your *sympathetic nervous system*, which governs your stress pathway through your fight-or-flight response. The really helpful thing is that these two systems are mutually exclusive; they can't be active at the same time. When the sympathetic system is dominant, you feel the effects of high stress. When the parasympathetic system is dominant, you feel calm. It's a see-saw effect because they both work in tandem. And the effects of each system are almost immediate.

Ryan and I did a number of deep breaths together, and then I taught him how to do the Stop–Breathe–Be technique and encouraged him to use it right before he went to meet with each radio producer.

Ryan's breathing calmed down over the phone. "That worked fast! Thank you! I'm adding that to my new Rule of 2."

Later that day I got a message from Ryan that his new breathing tools had worked beautifully and he had soared through his interactions with the people he had to meet that day.

Like Ryan, your stress will incrementally decrease over time through the strategies in this book. The tea kettle of stress is all about opening the valve and allowing your brain and body to slowly release the buildup of high stress. Opening up that therapeutic steam valve naturally decreases the fight-or-flight response of your sympathetic nervous system.

Dealing directly with the sympathetic nervous system can take some time. These breathing techniques work quickly because they leap over the sympathetic system and work directly on your parasympathetic system activity, helping you feel calmer, more present, and less stressed almost immediately, especially when you're actively feeling the negative effects of your maladaptive stress response. These breathing techniques can help you temporarily quiet your canary, whereas the rest of the techniques in this book can help you silence your canary for good.

4-7-8 Breathing

Once you've practiced the technique of diaphragmatic breathing, you can learn the more advanced breathing technique called 4-7-8 breathing.[4] I teach this technique to my patients and also use it myself. It is most effective when you're having trouble falling asleep or staying asleep. It's best done while lying down, because as a beginner you may feel some lightheadedness if you do it upright.

Follow the same guidelines you would for simple diaphragmatic breathing, using a slow and deep inhale and exhale:

1. Place one hand on your belly and the other hand on your chest. It doesn't matter which hand goes where. Feel your belly rise and fall with your breathing.

2. Inhale deeply through your nose for a slow count of 4.

3. Then hold your breath for a slow count of 7.

4. Finally, exhale through your nose or mouth for a slow count of 8.

5. Repeat this breath cycle two or three times, and then take a break and breathe normally with your natural breathing pattern.

6. Once you've rested and recalibrated, try the 4-7-8 breathing technique again for another two to three cycles.

Many of my patients say this is one of the most effective sleep-inducing aides they've used. The reason the 4-7-8 breathing technique is so effective is because it's based on the mind-body-breath connection. When you practice the 4-7-8 breathing technique, or even simple diaphragmatic breathing, you're intentionally activating your parasympathetic nervous system, and that has a direct effect on deactivating your sympathetic nervous system. This is why techniques like diaphragmatic and 4-7-8 breathing are so effective at resetting your stress from the inside out.

Heart-Centered Breathing

Another breathing technique that can help you when you're feeling depleted is called heart-centered breathing, and it works in similar ways, physiologically, to the other two techniques. But because you're placing your hand on your heart, it can feel self-soothing during particularly sad or despondent moments:

1. Put one hand on your heart and one hand on your belly. It doesn't matter which hand goes where. Feel your belly rise and fall with your breathing.

2. Inhale through your nose for a slow count of 4.

3. Exhale through your nose or mouth for a slow count of 7.

4. Do this for a few breath cycles until you're able to self-soothe.

When I've taught this technique to patients in the clinic, they tell me it helps them feel more connected to themselves in the moment with a greater sense of self-compassion. You can try it for yourself during emotionally depleting moments to see how it can help you cope and self-soothe, too.

Regardless of which breathing technique you use, your breath can serve as a powerful tool to activate and influence your mind-body connection for a life with less stress and more resilience.

When I was learning these breathing techniques, I came to appreciate this quote from the spiritual teacher Eckhart Tolle, who best described the impact your breath can have on your emotional state: "Be aware of your breathing as often as you are able, whenever you remember. Do that for one year, and it will be powerfully transformative . . . And it's free."[5]

Taking stock of your breathing at different points of your day can be a wonderful reminder of how connected your breath is to your mental state. When going about your day, take a few seconds to pay attention to your breath without interfering with it. Be the observer. Notice where you feel your breath—in your nostrils, in your chest or belly. Notice how it cycles in and out of your body at a specific cadence. This is your breath's natural rhythm. Familiarizing yourself with your natural breathing pattern helps to stimulate your mind-body connection into action.

Begin to incorporate these four techniques—Stop–Breathe–Be, diaphragmatic breathing, 4-7-8 breathing, and heart-centered breathing—into your daily life when you need to. In the early days, as I was learning to practice these methods, I'd put sticky notes with the words *STOP–BREATHE–BE* on my computer screen at work, the toothbrush holder in my bathroom, my laundry machine, and the electric tea kettle in my kitchen. These are four mundane moments that are ripe with the possibility of tapping into your mind-body connection to rewire your brain for less stress. As you start to pay attention to the mind-body-breath connection in your own life, you're going to start feeling better.

Grounding yourself through your breath during times of turmoil and stress helps you slow down your stress cascade and stay present and clear-headed in the moment. A sense of presence in the here and now, no matter the circumstance, is what a strong mind-body connection is all about!

Movement Decompresses a Stressed Brain

Remember from Chapter 1 my patient Miles, the manager of a software division, who was dismissive of his stress and had come to see me only at the insistence of his wife? Six months later, he came back to my office. And he had a different perspective this time.

Miles had faced a reckoning. His doctor had recently diagnosed him with high blood pressure and prediabetes. He had suggested that Miles start taking medication, but at Miles's insistence, his doctor agreed to wait two months to give him a chance to make changes to his lifestyle first. This time, Miles was here to see me not as a promise to his wife but as a way to stop his downward stress spiral for himself.

Of course Miles wasn't my first patient who had ignored how his stress negatively impacted his life. Coming to terms with your unhealthy stress is often the last resort for most people, once they've exhausted all other options. We've been so indoctrinated by hustle culture and the resilience myth that admitting to yourself that your runaway stress is influencing your health and adding to your symptoms can often feel like defeat. Yet, there is a relief to relinquishing the ongoing battle against yourself, knowing that it's a no-win situation unless you make changes. It's actually a sign of strength to choose to look at your mounting unhealthy stress and decide to take action even if you never imagined yourself in this position.

"Look, I can't go downhill like this," Miles told me, with trepidation in his voice. "I need to be healthy. I've got a family to take care of, kids to raise." I could tell he was not used to feeling emotionally or physically vulnerable, especially because he had been a Division I athlete in college.

"One minute I was this young hotshot athlete and the next minute I'm an out-of-shape, middle-aged corporate man who feels winded after a leisurely bike ride with my kids," Miles said incredulously. "I'm still in shock that my doctor wants me to start medication."

"It's not your fault, Miles" I reassured him. "Our everyday lives are designed to keep us sitting all day. You're not alone in this."

Data show that Americans are sitting more now than ever before, sometimes more than eight hours a day.[6] Although sitting too much seems like a passive and harmless thing to do, it can have real consequences on your health and well-being. A study of nearly eight hundred thousand people found that those who sat the most had a 112 percent higher risk of diabetes, a 147 percent higher risk of heart disease, a 90 percent higher risk of death from heart disease, and a 50 percent higher risk of death overall![7]

If you've heard the expression *sitting is the new smoking*, these findings highlight why. Too much sitting can be a risk for your physical health, but it can also be detrimental to your mental health. Researchers have found an association between too much sitting and your mood. Several studies show strong links between too much sitting and a higher risk of anxiety and depression.[8] "Sitting is a sneaky behavior," the researchers pointed out. "It's something we do all the time without thinking about it."[9]

Miles reflected on his own daily schedule. "You're right. I sit at my desk all day for work. Then I sit on the couch for a few hours at night. I don't even have to stand up to turn off a light or lower the heat. I can do it from my smartphone! Wow."

"Listen, I get it," I said. "Sometimes I text my husband even when he's in the next room! It's a lot faster, and less effort."

Miles laughed, but then looked serious. "You know, the longest I stand up might be in the shower and when I'm brushing my teeth. This has really been an eye-opener."

Miles took a shaky breath, and I could see his eyes begin to tear up a bit.

"Remember how I told you last time that my dad never missed work for a single day?" he said. "I always thought that was something to admire. He sat at his corporate job all day and then came home and sat at his desk in his home office. He thought about his job all the time, never even enjoying life. I never saw him sleep, either. He gained weight over time, just like I've been doing."

I said, "Those are good insights, Miles. I'm sure your dad did the best he could with the information he had at that time. But we know so much more now about how stress impacts the brain and body. Here's your chance to do the best you can with this new information available to you."

Miles was now recognizing that he couldn't "wait" to deal with his stress until he had the time. He had had a wake-up call at his doctor's office and felt a sense of urgency to take action and reset his stress.

"I guess I'll have to spring for a trainer or get back to the gym for ten hours a week," Miles said. "It's going to be rough."

"It doesn't have to be rough," I suggested. "Just a little bit of activity can make a difference. You can start by taking a little time every day to get out of your head and into your body. That's going to get your mind into a better place, too."

We discussed the benefits of the Rule of 2, and the first intervention I prescribed for Miles was a twenty-minute walk every day. He looked at me with skepticism. "No offense," he said, "but a twenty-minute walk isn't going to do much for me. I was an athlete. I know what it takes to lose twenty pounds. And besides, it's tough to find twenty free minutes in my day."

"Do you scroll through LinkedIn every day?" I asked.

He told me he spent about twenty minutes on LinkedIn a few times a day for his business, looking for new candidates with engineering degrees to possibly hire.

I prescribed an even swap. "Substitute one LinkedIn session with a walk instead," I suggested.

Miles shrugged his shoulders and grinned, "I mean, I'll do it because you want me to, but it's not going to work."

"It's going to be more stress for you to make a huge lifestyle overhaul, all of a sudden," I explained to Miles. "Let's start with two small, incremental changes that will end up being more effective and sustainable. Walking is the first one."

A Little Goes a Long Way

Like many of my patients, Miles believed that only long and intense sessions of hard exercise could improve his health. With little spare time to fit longer exercise sessions into his busy day, Miles forfeited physical activity altogether, even though he knew how important it was to his overall health.

Miles isn't alone in his all-or-nothing thinking. Even though 75 percent of people believe exercise is important for better health, only 30 percent get the recommended amount of exercise.[10] The exercise gap isn't about knowledge, it's about action.

We all know an exercise fanatic or two, but the majority of us have a tough time exercising regularly. Exercise equals dread for most of us. Creating an exercise habit is hard work. When you're depleted with stress, it seems like it takes a herculean effort. If you do push through the inertia and lace up your sneakers, you may have to face the mental and physical discomfort of starting out. You may have some soreness from using muscles that have been inactive for a while. You might feel uncoordinated or self-critical about how your body moves. You might not like the feeling that you've got too much ground to gain to feel like you accomplished anything. Even some of our greatest athletes don't like to exercise. Muhammad Ali, who held the heavyweight boxing championship title for many years, said, "I hated every minute of training. But I said, Don't quit. Suffer now and live the rest of your life as a champion."

While it's reassuring that even elite athletes don't like to exercise, the difference is that they do it anyway. They lean in to the idea that exercise requires discipline, while the rest of us lean in to the idea that exercise requires motivation. The truth is, no human being can be motivated to exercise every day. Nearly every patient I've ever asked about how they came to be regular exercisers have all said the same thing: "On the days I don't want to exercise, I think about how I'll feel after I'm done. Sometimes that's the only thing that can get me started."

Over the years, my patients have had real and legitimate barriers to exercise like a lack of time, energy, and motivation. But one of the greatest barriers I've witnessed in my patients (and myself) that no one ever verbalizes but everyone intrinsically feels is the all-or-nothing thinking when it comes to exercise. If we can't give it our all for a workout that day, then why bother trying in the first place?

We give ourselves so much leeway with other areas of our health, like sleep and diet, but we leave no space for imperfection when it comes to exercise. Imagine if you treated exercise like you do your sleep. You may struggle with getting enough sleep, delay it until the last possible minute, accept that it's not always going to be great, but you still try to get a little bit within a twenty-four-hour stretch of time. You wouldn't think, "I don't have time to get a full eight hours tonight, so why bother sleeping at all?" We accept imperfection in our sleep and are grateful when we can get a little shuteye when it's tough to come by. Why don't we give exercise the same grace?

Much of our all-or-nothing thinking for exercise originates from the tremendous value we've placed on the physical, aspirational aspects of exercise. These images and connotations of fitness—taut bellies and muscular physiques—feel so out of reach, and sometimes even triggering, that people who are legitimately trying to bring exercise into their lives after a long hiatus are often discouraged.

It's unfortunate that exercise is so closely linked to our society's fixation on weight loss and thinness, because studies show that the greatest benefits of exercise are all about improved overall fitness and well-being, not necessarily weight loss. Even without any changes to weight, adults who start exercising can improve their risk of worsening blood pressure, cholesterol, and diabetes.[11] Overweight adults who begin to exercise can reduce their risk of premature death by 30 percent with no change in weight.[12] The benefits of exercise for your brain and body far outweigh any changes on your scale. In fact, of the thousands of patients I've counseled in starting an exercise habit, not one has ever been motivated by the cosmetic promise of fitness. The tipping point for my patients has always been the mental promise: the many ways that exercise can change their stressed brains.

Miles was intrigued with the possibility of more mental fitness and better brain health.[13]

"Remember the tea kettle analogy?" I asked Miles. "Exercise can be a potent way to release therapeutic steam."

Exercising Your Stressed Brain

The neuroscientist Paul Thompson has studied thousands of brains to understand the links between brain health, stress, and exercise. "One theory is that it reduces stress," Thompson says. "We scanned [the brains of] people with high cortisol levels. If you're stressed, your cortisol levels can be very high. One of the things we found is that people with high cortisol levels lost brain tissue faster. That's a serious problem."[14]

Studies have confirmed Thompson's findings. Chronic stress can prematurely shrink your brain through chronically high levels of cortisol.[15] The good news is that brain shrinkage from too much stress is preventable and in some instances also reversible. Thompson offers us hope: "As soon as you know that's true, you can look at ways of reducing your cortisol. That's a very easy thing. We can get less stressed by exercising, walking, and taking breaks. There's a lot of ways that you can take care of your brain."[16]

While stress shrinks the size of your brain, exercise can help certain brain areas grow. Studies show that physical activity can thicken your prefrontal cortex and increase its connectivity and improve its function.[17] That's why, in part, exercise can help you have better problem-solving skills, attention, cognitive abilities, and memory.[18]

Even if you're a mostly sedentary person, like Miles, sitting at a desk for work for most of the day and driving to and from most places, you can still reap these brain changes if you exercise a little every day. In one study of thirty adults, people who exercised every day had a thicker prefrontal cortex compared with those who didn't.[19]

Another important role of your prefrontal cortex is communicating directly with your amygdala to help manage your stress response. Early brain research has found that exercise can also improve the connectivity between your prefrontal cortex and your amygdala.[20] With a larger, more connected, and smoother functioning prefrontal cortex, your brain is better equipped to handle life's stresses.

Another brain area that grows with exercise is the hippocampus, which is responsible for learning and memory (see Chapter 2). Studies show exercise is one of the few interventions that can grow new hippocampal brain cells, which has huge implications for your aging brain.[21] In fact, studies found that exercise may help reduce your risk of developing Alzheimer's dementia by almost 45 percent.[22]

Miles told me that his grandfather had died of Alzheimer's dementia and Miles had started monitoring his own memory for safe measure. If he could do something today to better protect his brain from stress and memory problems in the future, he wanted to. These brain benefits of exercise were his tipping point.

Miles agreed to free up twenty minutes each day (which is only 1.4 percent of his day) to build an exercise habit.

More and more scientific results are showing that even a few minutes of movement every day can benefit your brain and body in positive ways. One study found that just ten minutes of mild exercise could improve your brain, and in another, ten minutes of walking improved mood.[23] One key study followed 25,241 people who were nonexercisers for almost seven years and found that ultrashort bursts of exercise of only one to two minutes a few times a day, like running for the bus or taking stairs instead of an elevator, were associated with a lower risk of dying from cancer by 40 percent and dying from heart disease by almost 50 percent.[24] Even an occasional walk around the golf course has been associated with improved cholesterol levels.[25]

"Are you giving me a prescription to play golf every day?" Miles laughed. He had once been an avid golfer but hadn't played in several years.

"You should play golf whenever you have some time, but for now I just need you to take a twenty-minute walk around the block every day," I said.

Then I explained my rationale for this prescription. "This walk serves two key purposes," I said. "The first is for physical fitness. You need to acclimate your body to daily movement."

"I guess I do," Miles admitted, "especially since I haven't done much for two decades. It's been a long hiatus."

"More important, Miles, I want you to do it for your mental fitness. That's the second purpose," I said. "The twenty-minute walk will prime your brain circuitry to develop a new habit and become a springboard for more exercise in the future."

Exercise was important for Miles's body, but it was equally important for his brain. "What's good for your body is also good for your brain," I reminded him.

Do You Live in Your Head?

Most of us spend all day living in our heads without really inhabiting our bodies. We're neck-up people, which is why becoming aware of your mind-body connection initially feels so new. During stress, this feeling of living from the neck up can increase, as you may be consumed with your negative thoughts and not paying much attention to what's happening to your body—that is, until your canary shows up with a persistent physical symptom and forces your awareness of what's happening from the neck down. It's often frightening. Many of the physical feelings I had when my canary sang—quicker heartbeat, faster breath, feeling flushed—caught me off guard and scared me because I was living in my head and unaware of my body's response to stress.

One important aspect of a daily walking habit is that it familiarizes you with your body and its sensations when you're calm. Many of the same sensations you might experience during an acute stress response, like a quicker heartbeat or faster breathing, also occur as part of your normal physiology when you exercise. With a daily walking habit, you get an opportunity to become more accustomed to these sensations in a controlled, predictable setting, so when these same sensations happen during an unpredictable, stressful moment, you're not as taken aback by them. They become less frightening, which means you're more likely to have the presence of mind to act, through using the many techniques in this book, to slow down your stress response while it's happening in real time. A daily walk helps your mind and body become sensitized to what your heart and lungs might experience under a normal stress response.

Your daily twenty-minute walk is a perfect opportunity to help you get out of your head and into your body.

I wanted Miles to do just that, so I asked him to refrain from checking his phone during his walk. His walk was an opportunity for him to get familiar with his bodily sensations, a chance for him to have a brief moment of pause and reflection during his stressed and hurried day.

Because his attention would be fully focused on walking, he wouldn't be distracted by a phone meeting with a colleague or an email or text. He could reintroduce that possibility later, once he was familiar with how his body felt as he walked, and after his brain pathways for daily exercise were fully wired. For now, I asked him whether he could lean in to the experience of walking itself.

"I want you to really articulate your feet on the ground, feel the earth below them, as you walk," I told him. "Then I want you to notice your breathing when you're walking. And then just bring your attention to how your body moves and feels as you're walking." I added, "Consider this a type of movement meditation."

Miles laughed, "I've never meditated! I can't sit there and do nothing. I'm curious about this movement meditation though. My wife tried to learn to meditate and had a tough time. I'll share this with her, too. Maybe she can do her own movement meditation."

If Miles had pushed back on the idea of walking for walking's sake, I would've been fine with him taking a work call or listening to music or a podcast during the walk. But from my experience with patients, that can be a slippery slope. One minute you're taking a quick call, and the next you're crouching down midwalk to check and respond to email. Technology can quickly suck us back in, even when we have the best intentions. So when you're starting a new walking habit, limit your distractions and focus on just the walk.

At first, most of my patients resist this suggestion. Of course, I get it. We spend very little time away from our devices. Twenty minutes without technology can feel challenging. So I suggest that they, at the very least, walk without using their devices until the daily walk has become an everyday habit. In sixty days, when the habit is established, I tell my patients that they can use their phones during their walks, if they would like. Most of them respond that they would rather continue without their phone. Those twenty minutes a day have become valuable alone time without distractions. The device-free walks are something they looked forward to and want to keep doing.

TECHNIQUE #8: Take Twenty

1. Find a time when you can add a twenty-minute walk to your day—then start walking, maybe even today!

2. While you walk, pay attention to your body in motion. Focus on the connection of each foot on the ground as you move forward. Become more aware of how your breath moves in and out. Take your eyes off your phone and use them to observe your surroundings, both close by and at a distance.

3. Once back inside from your walk, add a checkmark to your calendar. Notice how calm yet invigorated you feel after your

short movement meditation. Capture that positive feeling and use it to motivate you for another short walk tomorrow. Keep your checkmark streak going every day, relishing your accomplishment of breaking through the inertia and getting your body in motion!

Breaking Through the Inertia

Starting a habit of a daily walk often feels like wading through molasses for many of my lifelong nonexercising patients. They're exhausted from their stress and living in their heads. Getting out of their heads and into their bodies is the last thing they want to do. It's just too much effort.

I remember during my own stress story, I was so overworked, sleep-deprived, and physically exhausted that the mere thought of going to the gym created a visceral negative reaction in me. It's not like I didn't try. There was a gym in the basement of my building, and I visited it a few times. I would walk in and see those large, overbearing machines and treadmills, look at myself in the gym's mirrored walls, and turn around to walk right back out. There was nothing welcoming or calming about that intense atmosphere when my body was running on empty.

My daily walking habit was something I stumbled into initially. One particularly nice evening, I left the hospital after a twelve-hour shift. The outside air felt refreshing. Instead of heading straight home, I took the scenic route around my neighborhood. I walked past my local coffee shop and headed down the block past my favorite small grocer, turned down restaurant row, and then took a lap around the perimeter of a nearby park before I went home and inside.

It was only an extra ten minutes, but I immediately sensed a change in my stress level. I enjoyed the sensation of moving my body for movement's sake—not to rush to deliver blood samples or lab specimens of a hospitalized patient but simply walking to walk. The next day, I did it again and added five more minutes. The day after that, I added five more. After the first three days, I walked every day the following week for twenty minutes each day. It became something I looked forward to, an enjoyable and relaxing way to end my day. It felt very different from my attempts at using the gym. When I got back to my apartment after my walk, my mind and body felt different—calmer, less hurried, and more present. I didn't know it at the time, but my brain was creating a neural pathway for walking. The feeling of reward, happening in my brain thanks to a few chemicals like dopamine, reinforced this pathway. I was creating a stress reset one walk at a time.

I broke through the inertia of sitting still, but it didn't happen overnight. It happened in slow, measured steps, incrementally. If you're stressed, you know well how the inertia of sitting still can keep you feeling stuck. It's like a gravitational force. You want to get unstuck but the thought of overcoming your inertia to move your body is utterly exhausting, so you put off exercise and keep sitting, which just makes you feel worse. It's a cycle.

If this is you, consider starting small. Aim for a walk around the block. If that feels good, walk around a little more the next day. The acts of making the decision to walk, getting dressed, heading outside, and feeling the fresh air on your face will help you feel better. When you're back inside from your walk, be sure to show yourself some compassion and congratulate yourself for breaking through the wall of inertia. Learn to celebrate your wins, big and small, on your stress journey.

"You want me to pat myself on the back after I take a walk?" Miles said smiling, looking incredulous.

"Yes I do. Your brain is changing every time you do something to reset your stress. That's worth celebrating," I reiterated.

The second prescription in my Rule of 2 for Miles had to do with the gut-brain connection (see more below) and beginning to make a small change in his eating habits. I suggested that instead of grabbing a donut in the break room at 10 a.m., Miles could choose some protein, such as a handful of almonds or sunflower seeds—something he could have ready to go that would be as easy as taking a donut.

As Miles was leaving my office, with one hand on the doorknob he turned around to me and said, "Our conversation reminded me of something my coach made me memorize in college: *Mens sana in corpore sano.* It's Latin for *a healthy mind in a healthy body.* Coach told us it was from the original Olympic games in ancient Greece. We laughed at him when he made us repeat it, but it really makes sense now." Miles left my office that afternoon and began his daily twenty-minute walk, which helped put his mind-body connection into action.

The Power of a Daily Habit

Miles knew that starting a new exercise habit every day would require effort, but he had a foolproof plan in place. Every new habit requires substantial amounts of mental bandwidth and brainpower initially, so your brain needs time to acclimate to the changes you're asking of it. The Rule of 2 and taking small steps help your brain to not register change as stress. Once your brain automates your new habit, it can become an everyday part of life.

The key to building new habits seamlessly into your life is making them easy, says writer Tara Parker-Pope. She describes it as reducing the friction of a new habit. Friction has three parts—time, distance and effort. To improve your chances of having a new habit stick, aim to decrease the friction associated with it.[26]

Miles had done this with his new plan, and the friction of his new habit was almost negligible. By swapping out an existing LinkedIn browsing session for a walk, he had overstepped time as a barrier. Because he wasn't traveling to a gym, distance wasn't an issue. Instead, he was going to take a break in his workday and take a short walk outside. We only had one more thing to address: the effort Miles would have to put in every day, even if that effort was small.

"Think of your daily walk like brushing your teeth," I explained. "It's a nonnegotiable commitment you're making with yourself. You do it whether you feel like it or not. Don't think about whether you want to or not; just lace up your sneakers and go."

Nearly every child and adult in America is trained from a very young age to brush their teeth every day. It's not something you decide to do, or ponder whether you have the time to do, or even say you'll skip today and do it extra tomorrow. It's automatic. As mundane and unpleasant as brushing your teeth can be, you just do it. Let's take a minute to consider how that happened from a brain science perspective.

Avoiding Decision Fatigue

Your brain circuit for toothbrushing was created when you were a child. We often don't think about brain circuits because many are created early in our lives, but we can learn a lot about habit formation through how we learned to brush our teeth every day. Your caregivers in childhood created a brain circuit for dental hygiene, and even though it can be a hassle, we continue with that habit as adults. Engaging in a daily walk helps your adult brain create a brain circuit for physical fitness hygiene.

When starting something new, it's easier for your brain to do it every day rather than once in a while. It avoids decision fatigue, which can easily set in no matter how committed you are initially. Think about the many times you've decided to start a new fitness regimen.

You enthusiastically say you'll go to the gym on Monday, Wednesday, and Friday. The first week, something comes up on Monday, so you tell yourself you'll go on Tuesday and Thursday. But you're delayed on Tuesday and can't make it. You commit to Wednesday and finally go. Then something comes up with your family on Thursday and then it's a busy weekend and you're back to Monday again. You've exercised a total of one day or maybe none, even though you had every intention of exercising multiple times your first week. This isn't about your limited willpower; it's about your biology of stress. The same brain machinery that powers new habit formation powers the stress mechanism in your brain. So when you're starting something new, start small and aim to do it every day.

This is why my exercise prescription always begins with a twenty-minute walk every day, because nearly everyone can do this, irrespective of their demands at work and at home. Once you've trained your brain and built the brain circuitry for an exercise habit, you can then add more intense gym sessions as often or as little as you'd like. The brain pathways have already been carved out through the daily walking regimen.

Sticking with Your Walking Habit

Once you've started your daily walking habit, you'll most likely feel a sense of accomplishment, which in turn will boost your enthusiasm. Let that enthusiasm carry you forward. Just be aware that your enthusiasm might wane after a few weeks. Your waning enthusiasm is a normal part of your biology and not a measure of your habit no longer being beneficial to your brain. In fact, it just means that you're moving into a new phase of habit formation and your brain is acclimatizing.

There are three phases to building a habit: the *initiation* phase when you start the habit, the *learning* phase when you repeat the habit, and the *stability* phase when the habit becomes automatic. The entire process takes on average about two months for most people. You should also expect a few hiccups, like missed days, along the way. These hiccups are part of your brain's learning process. Researchers confirm that "missing an occasional opportunity to perform the behaviour did not seriously impair the habit formation process . . . [but] unrealistic expectations of the duration of the habit formation process can lead [you] to give up during the learning phase."[27] Trust the process and let your brain take the full two months to solidify its new neural pathway. Even our brains need a little compassion from us while they're working hard to create a new habit. The science is clear: building a new habit, whether it's your daily walk or any other technique in this book, is about progress, not perfection.

When Miles came in for his follow-up a month later, we reviewed the checkmarks that showed how many days he'd walked the previous month. To his surprise, he had walked twenty-eight of the thirty days of that month! He was on his way to building an exercise habit. There were days when it was difficult for him to do the daily twenty-minute walk, but on those days he scheduled a walking meeting with a colleague or took a walk after dinner. Those still counted as checkmarks. Tracking his progress every day also gave him a sense of accomplishment and completion, which added to his motivation to continue his daily walking habit.

"I can't believe this little walk has made such a difference!" Miles told me. "I'm enjoying the fresh air, checking out the leaves changing color. I don't think I ever noticed the seasons before. I'm feeling more encouraged, and I can already tell that my mind feels sharper since I've been swapping out the mid-morning donut for a handful of almonds or walnuts. I never expected that."

"So, even though it's simple small changes, it's making a bigger difference," I said.

"It really is. Now I don't want to miss it. I need to get my walk in every day, no matter what. Even my assistant reminds me to get outside for my walk. And my fourth-grader puts a baggie of almonds in my briefcase every morning and one in his own lunchbox. So, he's learning a good daily habit, too."

Miles was on his way to creating a new brain circuit of daily movement and would soon reap all of the benefits for his brain and body that came with this new habit.

Through his daily walks, his stress improved, along with his sleep and energy. Eventually, he added three gym sessions a week and made more changes to his diet. When he saw his doctor for a follow-up in four months, his blood pressure was back in the normal range. He was still prediabetic but instead of starting medications right away, his doctor agreed to recheck blood work in another month and assess his need for medications at that time. Miles was determined to keep his progress going.

Bringing Movement into Your Life

I used to be a nonexerciser too, but one conversation with a ninety-two-year-old woman during my stress struggle changed my outlook on exercise. I went on a hiking trip to Darjeeling, India, at the foothills of the Himalayas. I wasn't a hiker or even a regular walker, so I stocked up on the latest gear—new jacket, boots, and backpack—thinking it would help. On my first day, as I struggled on a trail, an old woman breezed past me wearing nothing but a sari, a wool sweater, and a pair of flip-flops with socks.

Later, I saw her in town at her outdoor retail stall. "I remember you!" I said.

She had whizzed past me on the hiking trail because she was late to open her stall. She had owned her small business for the previous five decades.

I asked her what her secret was for being so physically and mentally agile at her age.

"You don't need that," she said pointing to my high-tech clothing and gear. "You need only this!" she said pointing to her head. "You can go anywhere with this!"

Since that day, whenever I think of a million excuses why I can't exercise, I remember the old woman's flip-flops and her mental fitness.

My excuses don't stand a chance.

In his 2008 book *The Blue Zone: Lessons for Living Longer from the People Who've Lived the Longest,* Dan Buettner describes the daily habits of the world's oldest living people. In terms of exercise, there's one big takeaway: those people don't do intense sweat sessions. They simply build low-intensity exercise into their everyday lives.

Given what you now know about how modern life encourages you to sit for most of your day and how just a little daily movement makes a big impact on your brain and body, consider how you can painlessly build some form of exercise into your life. How can you bring into your life some of this wise elder energy as you move through your day tomorrow? Instead of parking close to an entrance of a building, park a little farther away and walk an extra hundred yards. Rather than taking the elevator up one or two flights, take the stairs instead. If your subway or bus stop is close to home or work, get off one stop earlier and walk the rest of the way. These are a few of the opportunities you may have available to you in your everyday life that can help you make movement a habit. These small moments are ripe for a reset that quite literally gets you one step closer to less stress and more resilience. Whether your catalyst for starting to move more is your stress, anxiety, heart health, or longevity, let it inspire you into forward motion.

As you consider how to bring exercise into your life, think about this saying by another wise elder, the Chinese philosopher Lao Tzu: "Do the difficult things while they are easy and do the great things while they are small. A journey of a thousand miles must begin with a single step."

The Gut-Brain Connection

Exercise is a long-established way to reset your stress by activating your mind-body connection. A lesser known way to reset your stress is by activating your *gut-brain connection*. If you've never heard of the gut-brain connection, you're not alone. It's a relatively new scientific construct, and even those within the medical community are in the early stages of fully understanding how wide of a reach the gut-brain connection can have on your mental and physical health. So far, what we definitively know is that your gut doesn't just function to maintain your digestion; it plays a role in many other bodily processes, such as your mood, mental health, and even your stress. In this context, your gut refers to your small and large intestines, because that is where a lot of the action of the gut-brain connection happens.

Even if this is the first time you're learning about the science of the gut-brain connection, it's not the first time you've felt its effects in your body. You've been using its terminology for decades. If you've ever had gut-wrenching emotions, a pit in your stomach, a gut feeling, or felt butterflies in your gut, you've experienced your gut-brain connection firsthand.

The gut-brain connection can impact your stress because your gut and brain are closely tied to each other through a two-way information channel. Scientists sometimes refer to your gut as your second brain because your gut is sensitive to your emotional state. It is home to your body's second largest collection of nerve cells, or neurons, second only to your brain.[28] Your brain sends "top-down" signals to your gut, and your gut sends "bottom-up" signals back to your brain—called *cross talk*.[29] Gut-brain cross talk serves as a telephone operator, connecting your brain to your gut, and has been implicated in a wide array of physical and mental health conditions—from diabetes and Parkinson's disease to anxiety and depression.[30] As it turns out, your gut-brain cross talk may also influence your stress response.

Raina told me she had what she called "a nervous stomach." Raina explained, "The day before any work presentation, I'll have belly pain, nausea, and need to go to the bathroom a lot. I forget that this happens to me and convince myself that it's a stomach bug. But it's always stress, because when I finish the presentation, my symptoms vanish!"

For many people like Raina, their canary symptoms show up in their gut-brain connection as nausea, stomach pain, indigestion, bloating, or changes to their appetite and bathroom habits. If you experience any of these symptoms under times of stress, maybe you've ignored your canary, too.

Raina knew the pattern of her nervous stomach symptoms was related to stress, but she didn't know what to do about it next. "I try to do a better job of time management and relax the night before a presentation, but I can't seem to shake my symptoms. It's really uncomfortable," she admitted.

Unfortunately, many people like Raina who suffer from an imbalance in their gut-brain connection try to tolerate their discomfort alone and suffer in silence rather than seek medical attention. If you suspect that your gut-brain connection symptoms might be related to stress, it's important to see your doctor to ensure that they aren't caused by an underlying medical condition. Even if you suspect that your stomach issue isn't due to stress, open communication with your doctor is key. There's a growing awareness of the gut-brain connection in conventional medical care, and many medical practices have links to psychologists with expertise in this field. Your doctor can help you navigate the complex medical system to get you the support and resources you need to heal, irrespective of the underlying reason.

When Raina came to my office, she had already seen her general physician, who had referred her to a gastroenterologist. After a thorough workup, Raina was diagnosed with irritable bowel syndrome (IBS). She had started treatment with her doctors. In addition to her treatment, her doctor suggested she could do a better job managing her stress.

"I understand that stress is worsening my symptoms, but having spa days isn't helping," she said. Raina was exasperated. "I need to figure out how to actually lower the stress in my body."

I understood and empathized with Raina's stress struggle, remembering my own well-meaning doctor's suggestion to just "relax more."

Raina had tried, unsuccessfully, to manage her stress on her own. She came to my office with the hopes of getting a concrete plan to help figure out how to respond to her canary's warnings. She was doing what most people do when they recognize their canary. She was managing her stress in the short term the day before a presentation. But then she'd go back to her normal routine once her acute stress episode was over. That normal routine consisted of late nights, irregular eating, and a nightly habit of drinking half a bottle of wine to decompress.

"It's great that you're making changes to your routine when your stress flares up," I reassured her, "but our goal together is to prevent, or at least to minimize, the frequency of flares in the first place."

Raina was caught in a familiar loop. Her stress would flare in the short term, forcing her to put her full attention into managing it. But once her acute stress period was over, she wouldn't pay much attention to her canary song or how her daily habits were contributing to her stress. A month would go by and everything would be fine. Then an inevitable presentation would come up, which was Raina's stress trigger, and her canary would sing out an alarm again.

Raina needed help breaking the cycle of stress. "Managing stress is a long game," I explained to her. "We're going to focus on making small, sustainable changes, two at a time, so that you can do them every day, not just before a big presentation."

The focus for Raina's Rule of 2 was to slowly and incrementally release some therapeutic built-up steam from her tea kettle of stress. We agreed to two key interventions: first, to protect her sleep by aiming for an earlier bedtime, and second, to make time for a daily twenty-minute walking reset.

In addition to our two interventions, Raina agreed to begin acupuncture, which studies have found helpful for IBS and other conditions related to the gut-brain connection.[31] She was also going to begin psychotherapy, which her primary doctor had prescribed. I encouraged her to discuss with her therapist the possibility of her being reliant on alcohol.

"I think you may be self-medicating with alcohol," I suggested, "It's something that people with high stress can often do."

"Wine definitely takes the edge off and helps me cope with my stress better," she admitted. "But it's not helping me achieve my long-term stress goals. I'd really like to figure out how to stop drinking every day."

Self-medicating with alcohol is a common phenomenon, especially among people with elevated stress.[32] Awareness and seeking professional help are critical and important first steps. I congratulated Raina on her willingness to explore her coping strategies and her readiness to make a change in her life.

Within the first three months of Raina starting her comprehensive treatment plan with her team of physicians, as well as putting her Rule of 2 into practice, her gut-brain connection symptoms dramatically improved. When she started to pay attention to her canary's warnings and make changes that supported her long-term stress goals, her canary quieted down. There was little doubt that Raina's canary had been her gut!

Researchers around the world are trying to understand how the gut-brain connection works so that they can determine how various therapies can benefit patients like Raina. "Our two brains 'talk' to each other," says Johns Hopkins physician Jay Pasricha, who studies the underpinnings of the gut-brain connection. "So therapies that help one may help the other . . . Psychological interventions [like therapy] may also help to 'improve communications' between the big brain and the brain in our gut."[33]

Your Gut as a Gateway to Managing Your Stress

This growing body of research suggests that your gut could soon be considered a potent gateway to help manage your stress. One of my early mentors would often say, "Why do we glorify the brain when it comes to stress? We need to do more to bring attention to the gut, because we know that's where things can happen!"

My professor was referring to the fact that 95 percent of your body's serotonin is found in your gut, and there are three to five times more serotonin receptors in your gut than in your brain.[34] Serotonin is a brain chemical, also known as a neurotransmitter, that's partly responsible for managing your mood. You've probably heard of serotonin in the context of the popular class of drugs called selective serotonin reuptake inhibitors (SSRIs), such as Prozac, which are used to improve mood and treat depression. Isn't it interesting that we refer to serotonin as a brain chemical when most of it is found in the gut? The gut truly is the second brain!

Understanding how to influence your gut-brain connection can be a useful tool in helping you minimize your stress. It helps to have some clarity on how stress can impact your gut-brain connection and vice versa.

Your gut is home to the largest microecosystem of healthy bacteria and other organisms in your body, called the *microbiome*.[35] This microbiome serves as a key intermediary in the information channel and cross talk between your gut and your brain. Even though these healthy bacteria live in your gut, they're involved in many functions in your body besides digestion such as immunity, mood regulation, stress management, and hundreds of other bodily functions.

Just like your brain changes and responds to stimuli through neuroplasticity, your gut microbiome can also alter its functions based on what's happening in your body. Many factors influence your gut microbiome, including your age, recent illnesses, medications, and especially stress. Periods of prolonged chronic stress can have an impact on your microbiome, changing its structure and composition so it's less robust.[36] While your gut microbiome is strengthened by many of the strategies offered in this book, like better sleep, less stress, and more exercise, it can be depleted through behaviors like smoking, drinking too much alcohol, not getting enough exercise, and sleeping poorly.

Recent studies have shown that within these trillions of healthy organisms that make up your gut microbiome there are specific bacteria whose sole function is to regulate your mood. This subset of bacteria within your gut microbiome is called the *psychobiome*, and these are the seat of your gut-brain connection when it comes to your mental health.[37] Scientists are working to uncover exactly how the psychobiome works to influence how we think and feel.

"What probably happens is that our brain and our gut are in constant communication," says John Cryan, a scientific researcher who studies medications that target the psychobiome. Cryan's colleague Gerald Clark adds, "It will be important to understand better and more precisely the mechanisms at play."[38]

Though the science is still new on how to specifically influence your psychobiome, we have enough data to suggest that your overall microbiome can be influenced by your habits and behaviors in the same way your brain is influenced by your daily actions through neuroplasticity. You can actively strengthen your overall microbiome to reset your stress and reverse your burnout through the many techniques I've already described in this book and those that are upcoming in the following chapters. In the same way that every technique can be a reset for your brain and stress, these techniques can also become helpful resets to get your overall gut microbiome to a healthier place.

Besides using your daily behaviors to influence your gut-brain connection, the microbiome is sensitive to what you eat. Studies show that certain foods can directly impact your microbiome.[39] In fact, the emerging field of *nutritional psychiatry* is focused primarily on how foods can affect your mental health, and its foundations lie in the gut-brain connection.[40]

Nutritional psychiatry can help guide you in choosing foods that can improve your stress. We'll cover those in the next section, but your everyday experience has probably already taught you something valuable about the interplay between stress and food.

For instance, you've probably noticed how stress can make you choose certain foods over others. When you're stressed, you may crave high-fat or high-sugar foods. This phenomenon is called *stress eating* or *emotional eating*, and it's exceedingly common. Enter the chocolate cake, the drive-thru French fries, the pint of ice cream, and the donut. Or in my case, blue corn tortilla chips, which have become my go-to guilty pleasure during stressful times—and I'm not talking about one serving size of eleven chips.

During stressful times, my patients say that they feel like they have no willpower to resist such foods. We see TV ads sending us strong messages that carefree, relaxed times come with a bag of chips, a can of soda, or a pint of ice cream. You don't see many people in TV commercials touting the benefits of a better life with a bag of baby spinach, right?

But there's an even deeper reason for our stress cravings for sugar, salt, and fat that predates television, going all the way back to that little lizard brain we've had since our cave dweller days. During periods of stress, our brains are biologically programmed to crave high-fat, high-sugar foods because these are the most calorically dense. As we've seen, when the amygdala, that little reptilian part of our brain, is activated during stress, we focus on survival. In the most literal of terms, calories equal survival. Your reptilian brain can't distinguish between stress caused by paying bills or stress caused by a famine, so you'd better bulk up your body while you can.

When you reach for your comfort food, it's because your brain is responding to your internal cues. But instead of berating yourself, as so many of us do, start by giving yourself some self-compassion and ask yourself this question posed by Deepak Chopra instead: What am I really hungry for?[41] Maybe it's more rest, certainty about the future, or more connection. Aim to give *that* to yourself, instead.

What Are You Hungry For?

"I've been getting by, day to day, with emotional support from friends," my new patient Lauren told me. Then she paused, laughed a little, and added, "And a whole lot of chocolate cake."

At age forty-nine, Lauren was twenty-two years into an intense full-time career in social work. Outside of her job, Lauren had the constant activities and concerns of her two teenage daughters, who were trying to become more independent, and a husband who had his hands full and put in long hours with his car dealership. Lauren's parents had moved nearby when the children were little to help out, but now they both had their own health issues and depended on Lauren for help with their needs.

"My anxiety isn't new to me," Lauren told me. "I've been seeing a therapist for about seven years. But my stress eating has gotten to a whole new level. I've gained almost twenty pounds in the past two years! My chocolate cake fix is backfiring."

Even though Lauren was trying to be light-hearted about it, I could tell by the way she twisted her hands on her lap that she was hitting a wall.

When I asked her to describe her pattern of emotional eating, she explained, "It started out as an occasional bedtime treat. But now, I can't let a day go by without indulging in chocolate cake. And the worst part is, I eat it right before bedtime, and the serving sizes have become bigger over time."

Lauren's face flushed with embarrassment. "I'm weak. I can't seem to curb this bad habit."

"First of all, you are far from weak, Lauren," I assured her. "You're overscheduled, you have an intense career, and you have loved ones who depend on you, so it makes sense that you're eating as a way to cope with your life's stresses."

Lauren replied, "But my circumstances aren't going to change anytime soon. So, then what?"

"You're right," I said. "Your chronic stress isn't going to magically disappear, which is why we're going to start with the Rule of 2."

As the first step, Lauren committed to a daily exercise program, beginning with a brisk twenty-minute walk every day. Exercise served two purposes for Lauren: to directly affect her anxiety and stress through the brain mechanisms we've discussed above, and to indirectly influence her prefrontal cortex—the part of your brain responsible for food cravings. Studies show that increased activity in the prefrontal cortex can help minimize food cravings, and exercise may help to modulate this pathway.[42]

In one study of fifty-one women, a brisk twenty-minute walk with an average speed of 3.5 miles per hour was found to help control food cravings for both chips and chocolate, resulting in less consumption of these foods. Researchers said that their findings "demonstrated that a bout of moderate aerobic exercise could both enhance inhibitory control [by the brain] and improve dietary choice [by the individual]."[43] This study, along with several others, shows us that exercise doesn't only help your body manage stress; it can also be a potent driver of changing your relationship to food cravings during stress.

The second part of Lauren's Rule of 2 was to start keeping a food log. Tracking what you eat and when can have a profound effect on your awareness of how much you eat. It has been shown to be one of the most effective weight-management tools. With Lauren's recent weight gain, she was eager to get a better handle on her eating overall, and specifically her chocolate cake fix, but it had been hard to do on her own. A food log would help her understand her eating patterns, and awareness is always the first step to making a change.

To show Lauren how powerful a food log can be, I shared the findings of a landmark study which showed that keeping a food log doubled people's weight loss.[44] Of the 1,685 participants, those who kept a food log lost more than twice the amount of weight than those who didn't. The small act of writing down what you eat throughout the day can have a big impact.

Lauren was encouraged by these findings. She was open to tracking her food intake, and since it didn't add to her existing anxiety, we included this in her Rule of 2. We also discussed how she could swap out chocolate cake for food that was more nutrient-dense and less calorically dense when she felt compelled to eat a bedtime snack. She agreed to try apples with peanut butter. "I'll need the sweetness and crunch of apples with the creamy, decadent texture of peanut butter," she said.

This prescribed Rule of 2 for Lauren was based on the premise that helping her manage her underlying stress and anxiety would then have a ripple effect on her emotional eating and she could make progress toward her long-term health goals.

Lauren now had a plan in place and was eager to implement it that very evening. When I checked back with her four weeks later via email, she said the plan was working, in spite of her full and overscheduled life. "I'm really enjoying my walking time and being alone," she told me. "It's the quiet time for myself I've been craving. It almost feels meditative for me, a nice break in my day. I've been going every single day, rain or shine. And I've increased my walking time from twenty to forty-five minutes. I'm learning these new coping skills so I'm less likely to reach for my chocolate cake!"

I encouraged Lauren to keep going.

When I saw her for a follow-up two months later, her Personalized Stress Score had dropped from 18 to 8. She shared her food log with me and was averaging bedtime eating only twice a week—a vast improvement from seven days a week! She had also gradually lost seven pounds. Lauren was in a much better place than when she had begun her stress journey a few months before.

As she was leaving my office, Lauren asked me what else she could do. She had built up momentum and wanted to keep it going. "I've gotten my Rule of 2 down. It's really working for me," she said proudly. "But I'm ready to take that next step. What else can I do with my diet to protect my health?"

In addition to continuing her daily brisk walking and food tracking, I suggested that Lauren begin to slowly incorporate the *Mediterranean Diet* into her life. She was intrigued when I explained the many health benefits of the Mediterranean Diet and was ready to bring some of its elements into her eating habits.

The Gold Standard of Eating for Better Health

When it comes to the links between stress and what you eat, the relationship goes both ways. Stress can make you crave certain types of foods, like chocolate cake for Lauren or blue corn tortilla chips for me. But certain foods can influence your levels of stress too. A wealth of information is available through the many studies in nutritional psychiatry on which foods to choose. But my patients tell me that even if they're interested in eating better, it's hard to keep up with the latest "superfoods." They're often frustrated with the changing trends.

When they ask me about the best diet to eat for less stress and better health, like Lauren did, I always recommend the Mediterranean Diet. The Mediterranean Diet is less of a strict diet and more of a general way of eating. Its focus is mostly on eating fresh fruits and vegetables, whole grains, legumes and beans, monounsaturated fats from nuts and olive oil, fish and chicken, and some dairy. There's no specific formula for eating a Mediterranean Diet, like other more prescriptive diets; it's more about combining these nutrient-dense, minimally processed foods into balanced meals. Compared with the standard American diet, the Mediterranean Diet overall includes eating fewer processed foods, less red meat, and fewer simple carbohydrates and saturated fats.

Of any diet, the Mediterranean Diet has been shown again and again, through hundreds of studies comparing different types of diets, to be the gold-standard way of eating for many common conditions and for overall health. It's been found to help with maintaining brain health, improving longevity, controlling weight, managing diabetes, and preventing chronic illnesses, including cancer.[45] It's also been shown to help mental health conditions like anxiety and depression. In one study, eating a modified Mediterranean Diet for three months reduced participants' self-reported anxiety symptoms.[46] In another, eating a Mediterranean-inspired diet rich in fruit, vegetables, fish, and lean meat was linked to fewer depressive symptoms.[47]

And since we're talking about the gut-brain connection, the Mediterranean Diet can also influence your microbiome. In a yearlong study across five European countries, participants following the Mediterranean Diet experienced improvements in their gut microbiome.[48]

Another important part of the Mediterranean Diet is its focus on prebiotic and probiotic foods, which has been built into the way of eating for centuries in many parts of the world. Both of these types of food can directly affect the gut microbiome to strengthen your gut-brain connection. *Prebiotic foods* include things like whole grains, oats, apples, bananas, onions, artichokes, garlic, asparagus, and even cocoa; these foods help feed the healthy gut bacteria in your microbiome. *Probiotic foods* are usually fermented foods and include things like yogurt, sauerkraut, kefir, and kombucha, which give back some healthy bacteria to your microbiome.[49]

While this way of eating is generally beneficial to prevent many chronic conditions, it's also an important consideration when it comes to managing your stress. One study found that increasing vegetable intake, as the Mediterranean Diet suggests, could help improve levels of perceived stress.[50] In another study of forty-five people, a diet rich in prebiotic and fermented foods decreased stress by 32 percent, and those participants who followed the diet more accurately had an even greater reduction in their stress.[51]

With the plethora of health benefits of a Mediterranean Diet, you may wonder how to bring this way of eating onto your plate. If you're currently eating the standard American diet and are curious about gradually adopting a new way of eating inspired by the Mediterranean Diet, here are a few simple swaps and choices you can make:[52]

- Add a rainbow of fruits and vegetables to your meals. Aim for five servings every day. Be sure to include some prebiotic vegetables in the rotation, such as mushrooms, green peas, legumes, and onions.
- Start using extra virgin olive oil as your cooking oil.
- Instead of red meat, eat fish or chicken and start eating more beans and legumes for protein.
- Swap out white bread for whole grain breads. Incorporate whole grains, too, such as oats and barley.
- Drink water instead of soda or juice.
- Add a few spoonfuls of probiotic foods like yogurt or sauerkraut to your weekly meals.

Like any life change, making changes in what you eat can add to your stress. So follow the Rule of 2 for incorporating the Mediterranean Diet into your life: make only two small changes at a time, and every few weeks, add two more. You will slowly and gradually cook and eat your way to better health.

As you begin to eat this new way, you're going to have to start shopping for food in a different way too. One technique I recommend to my interested patients, and one I use myself, is to shop the perimeter of your grocery store. Most supermarkets have the same setup: the center aisles have boxed, processed, and calorically dense foods, while the perimeter has fresh, minimally processed, and nutritionally dense foods that are close to their natural state. There's a produce section, grain section, protein section, and dairy section. By shopping the perimeter of your grocery store, your food choices will slowly start to mimic the Mediterranean Diet with minimal effort.

TECHNIQUE #9: Let Your Gut Lead the Way

Most of us grew up enjoying certain foods and thinking that if a grocery store sells it, it must be healthy enough. We now know that many of the foods sold in stores are made for convenience and a long shelf life, rather than what's best for the body. Here are some simple ideas for checking in with what would make your gut happy and boost your brain, too:

- Keep a log of what you eat during an average day, especially noting the foods you consume when you're feeling stressed. Many of us crave high-fat, high-sugar foods when stressed.

- The next time you go to the grocery store, make a choice to walk the outer perimeter first and fill up your grocery cart with fresh food items before shopping the inner aisles where more of the processed and preserved foods are displayed.

- Every week, aim to incorporate one or two additional foods from the Mediterranean Diet list.

- If you go to the fridge or cupboard to get a snack even when you're not hungry, pause to check in with why you crave a snack. Perhaps you really want a break from your workday, or a change of scenery. Maybe you need to have a moment of self-compassion because you're facing something that makes you uncomfortable. Or it could be simple boredom that can't be solved with a peanut butter cup.

Emotional eating is part of our biology. Learn to decipher your body's signals for hunger from your body's reaction to boredom, frustration, anger, worry, and the many other emotional reasons we eat when we're not hungry. Your stress will thank you for knowing the difference.

Three months after I first saw her, Lauren sent me an email with this subject headline: "Good News!" She had lost eleven pounds with the three techniques she had put into place. Through taking her brisk twenty-minute daily walk, keeping a food log, and eating more of a Mediterranean Diet, Lauren had made major strides in her stress, weight, and gut-brain connection. Besides the mere number on the scale, Lauren felt a great sense of achievement for what she had been able to do with a few simple techniques using her Rule of 2 in just over three months. This confidence carried over into other areas of her life. Her co-workers noticed and so did her family.

"Everyone has been asking me what I've been doing. It's not just how I look, but more important, how I feel," Lauren said. "I felt out of control before, but these small steps have helped me feel in control of my life again."

Lauren had found a way, through her Rule of 2, to slow down her runaway stress in spite of nothing else changing in her external environment. She still had the same challenges at home and at work, but she was able to better manage those life stresses. Lauren's success was due to her progress, not to perfection.

Lauren needed something to help her self-soothe and cope with difficult emotions. Food is a great pleasure of life meant to be enjoyed. It wasn't realistic to expect a zero-chocolate-cake policy. By addressing Lauren's emotions gently and with compassion, through an exercise program, food log, and gradual dietary changes, she was able to reset her stress. Lauren had learned to sync her brain and her body.

Raina's and Lauren's stories may seem to be overnight successes to you, but in reality, both women required many small, slow, and incremental steps (along with plenty of missteps!) on their paths. Syncing your brain and your body to strengthen your mind-body connection is a skill that takes practice. But with the four techniques in this reset—learning how to be present with Stop–Breathe–Be, recalibrating your stress response using the demonstrated breathing techniques, moving your body a little every day to get out of your head, and leading with your gut—you too can become your own success story soon enough. It just takes a little practice to get there.

6

The Fourth Reset: Come Up for Air

"Nothing I do is good enough. No matter how hard I work, my productivity is worse than it's ever been!" Holly explained, waving her hands around. "I'm working harder than ever to just stay in place. I'm completely drained at the end of every day. It's like I can't come up for air!"

Considering the high percentage of people who are suffering from burnout, I know Holly isn't the only one feeling like she's giving it her all but only staying in place.

"I've worked in the tech industry for seventeen years," she said. "I used to be the one who had it all going on. But with artificial intelligence on the rise, I'm worried about the many rapid changes. If I fall behind at work, my position might be outsourced to an A.I. program."

Holly was a high achiever—a graduate of MIT with a track record of having an illustrious tech career. But recently, she has been stuck in a pattern of high stress and low productivity. I assured Holly that the stress and burnout she was feeling weren't the exception, but the rule. "Your concerns are valid. It's the new normal, and the old rules don't apply," I said. "But A.I. can't provide the irreplaceable human factor that you bring to work every day."

"I know," Holly sighed. "My company appreciates me and my expertise. There just aren't enough hours in the day to keep up with all the rapid changes."

"No one can keep up the pace and stay in the race without also taking a break," I sympathized. "Even marathon races have a finish line, but our work and home lives don't. So we have to create some time to catch our breath."

Holly had been running on empty for the previous few years. She knew she was experiencing burnout, yet she held herself to the same high-functioning standards of productivity she had before her burnout set in.

Like many of my patients, Holly was taught at a young age how to put others' needs before her own, so paying attention to her canary symptoms required a change in perspective. Maybe you're experiencing something similar to what Holly is going through. If so, you might be thinking, "How can I reset from burnout when I'm doing the best I possibly can and it's still not helping?"

In this Fourth Reset, Come Up for Air, you'll learn the mechanics of how you can give your brain a breather without sacrificing your productivity. In fact, the techniques in this reset may help you enhance your productivity, even in the midst of your stress and burnout. Through the three techniques offered here, you'll be able to do less to achieve more, create healthy boundaries to maintain your energy and focus, and feel more in control as you juggle your many roles at work and at home.

Even if your stress feels overwhelming, irrespective of your current circumstances, the Fourth Reset will help you find mental space so your brain can gradually recalibrate to its optimal functioning. As the science shows, your brain functions best when it's not overloaded, which is why the Rule of 2 has a high success rate. So keep the Rule of 2 in mind as you learn the three techniques in this Fourth Reset: the Goldilocks Principle, the Magic of Monotasking (or the Myth of Multitasking), and the Fake Commute.

The Goldilocks Principle

How could aiming to be like Goldilocks have a positive effect on your level of stress? Because that little girl with golden hair, even under the threat of angry bears, was able to find the "just right" way to take care of herself.

If you've been feeling stressed and burned out recently, it's more than likely that your productivity has suffered. You're not functioning at the top of your game in any sphere of your life. You're barely surviving and certainly not thriving. Your internal self-talk may be pushing you to work harder and faster to catch up to your old productivity standards, but this just slows you down and makes you less productive.

Holly was living the resilience myth, so for her Rule of 2, my first suggestion was for her to do less at work and make her breaks count. Her eyes narrowed and she visibly scoffed at my suggestion. Doing less had never been an option for her. But with her increasing burnout and stress, she was feeling that she had run out of options. "Obviously, what I'm currently doing isn't working," she said.

Holly decided she was ready to embrace a new way to work. I assured her that this first prescription of doing less in the short term would allow her to achieve far more in the long term.

"You may believe that stress impacts the brain and body in a straight, linear way," I explained, drawing a graph on paper, with a line in an upwards slope. "The more stress, the worse off you are, right?"

Holly nodded. "That sounds about right."

"But actually, research has shown that our stress response is like a bell-shaped curve," I clarified.[1] "When you have too little stress in your life, you're on the left side of this curve. This shows up as you being bored, unmotivated, and unproductive. But on the flip side, when you have too much stress, which is where you are, you're on the right side of the curve. You feel anxious, depleted, and unproductive."

I continued: "Right in the middle of the curve is your sweet spot for stress—not too much and not too little when your stress is just right. This is your healthy stress level where you feel motivated but not overwhelmed, engaged but not depleted.[2] In this sweet spot of stress, your brain and body function optimally. This is called your body's *adaptive response to stress*."

What I had described to Holly was what I call the Goldilocks Principle of stress.

It's probably safe for me to assume that, like Holly, you are also on the right side of the curve right now with too much stress and possibly burnout. Our work together is to help you gradually shift from being on the right side of the curve with too much stress, to somewhere in the middle, that is, the top of the bell curve, near your sweet spot of healthy stress.

The remedy for getting to your sweet spot of stress is, of course, slowing down and doing less. But with demanding bosses and approaching deadlines, that's the farthest thing from reality.

You may be thinking that the Goldilocks Principle is great in theory, but it's not realistic or practical in your life. You don't think you can slow down and do less at work without everything falling apart or finding yourself getting fired.

I understand. Goldilocks herself, in the story, was actually trespassing in the bears' home and not facing the reality of her life. She didn't last long, pretending a different life was hers.

You have real-world obligations to uphold, like working your job; paying your bills, a monthly mortgage, or rent; and maintaining relationships. You don't have the luxury of scaling back until your stress level hits your sweet spot and is "just right."

As much as we'd all love to step away from our responsibilities and head to a beach in Bali, I want to give you the real-world application of the Goldilocks Principle: honor your breaks.

"Instead of going right from one meeting to the next, I want you to take a short break between meetings," I suggested to Holly.

Because Holly loved data, I shared a study conducted by Microsoft that compared brain scans of people who were in back-to-back meetings with brain scans of people who took short breaks. The study found that the brain scans in the group taking short breaks showed significantly less stress. Short, frequent ten minute breaks decreased the cumulative effects of work stress on the brain.[3] This helped Holly become more enthusiastic about honoring her breaks.

If you're like Holly, you probably do what we all do between meetings and work tasks: you scroll mindlessly through social media or quickly glance at your email inbox. Instead, as part of your Fourth Reset, spend your break time intentionally working on your stress: do some gentle stretches at your desk, get up and take a quick five-minute walk, or practice the relaxation and breathing techniques you learned in Chapter 5. Aim to begin building your new habit of staying intentional and present during your breaks so you can gradually shift your stress levels from the right side of the curve back toward the middle near your sweet spot.

It's like the tea kettle analogy—find ways to blow off therapeutic steam.

By honoring your breaks, rather than spending them mindlessly in activities that might promote stress, you can achieve the Goldilocks Principle of "just right" stress in theory and in practice!

When Holly understood where she was on her stress curve and

compared it with where she wanted eventually to be, she started to put the Goldilocks Principle into practice by honoring her breaks. Working in tech meant she spent most of her day on a computer and in meetings. Between meetings Holly began stepping away from all tech screens, including her phone, to stand up and stretch and do some deep breathing. Once a day she took a brisk walk to get herself into a better mindset. If an outdoors walk wasn't possible, Holly would head to the stairwell in her building and go up and down a couple flights of stairs for ten minutes. Her co-workers thought she was on her way to another meeting.

"It takes at least eight weeks to build a habit," I reminded Holly, "so find ways to make these changes automatic."

To help her brain create a new habit, Holly scheduled several three-to-five-minute blocks into her work calendar immediately after long meetings and peppered them throughout the day. Because they were small increments of time, none of her co-workers or her assistant seemed to notice. She committed to honoring her breaks for two months, and with time and patience, her stress levels gradually drifted to a lower, healthier state. When she compared her Personalized Stress Score from her first visit to her score two months later, she saw a ten-point reduction. She said she felt that change in her daily life. Holly had found her sweet spot of stress by honoring her breaks in spite of working in a fast-paced environment. She was figuring out how to come up for air in the midst of her fast-paced work life.

TECHNIQUE #10: Follow the Goldilocks Principle for "Just Right" Stress

Find the natural breaks in your daily schedule, which could be when you switch from one task to another, when you are leaving a meeting, when you are between classes, when you finish a section of a longer project, etc. Instead of checking your smartphone or hurrying on to what's next, choose to take three to five minutes to give your mind time to reset.

During your short break, unite your mind with your body through a physical action: stand up and stretch, look out a window as you do some diaphragmatic breathing, take a short walk in the hallway, or go up and down some stairs. Stay present with the way you feel physically in the moment instead of letting your thoughts race ahead to what's next on your list.

1. Move toward integrating five or six short breaks of three to five minutes into your day.

2. Make this a daily practice for three months and observe whether your productivity increases and your stress minimizes.

The Goldilocks Principle helps to debunk a common productivity myth in our hustle culture that working faster, harder, and longer is the only way to improve productivity. That is a scientific fallacy and couldn't be farther from the truth. Your brain works better and more efficiently, especially when you're managing new tasks, if it's given time to decompress. Honoring your breaks not only can lower your stress in the short term, but it can fuel your productivity in the long term.

Taking breaks can help you build a better functioning brain. When you step away from a task you're working on, you're letting your brain and its neural pathways go through an important process called *consolidation*.

Neural consolidation is when new learning and information that's been floating around in your head gets cemented into pathways and circuits for future use. A study looked at brain scans of twenty-seven healthy adults and found that even a short, ten-second break improved learning through consolidation.[4] When the researchers compared these healthy brain scans, they found that the brains changed more during rest than during learning sessions.[5]

This prompted the researchers to investigate when the learning was actually happening—during practice or during rest? "Everyone thinks you need to 'practice, practice, practice' when learning something new," said the study's senior author, Leonardo G. Cohen. "Instead, we found that resting, early and often, may be just as critical to learning as practice."[6]

Holly laughed when I shared this study's findings with her. "That happened to me last week!" she exclaimed. "I had spent hours huddled over my computer at night trying to solve a tech problem for work. I couldn't figure out what was wrong so I gave up and started getting ready for bed. I was in the shower and then it suddenly dawned on me what the glitch was! And I was able to fix it the next morning!"

"You gave your brain a breather and had a breakthrough," I confirmed.

Like Holly, you're more capable of having your own breakthroughs with a little help from short, intentional breaks. And they need to be only ten seconds long to be worthwhile for your brain.

Multitasking Is a Myth

The second intervention in Holly's Rule of 2 was to minimize her multitasking. She was a self-proclaimed "excellent multitasker" and wore this badge with pride. "Being a great multitasker got me promoted quickly," Holly said. "I used to be able to do four things at once. But now my energy is dragging, everything takes me twice as long, and I'm making mistakes more often. I probably need to slow down."

The data match Holly's experience. Eighty-two percent of American workers say they multitask every day, more than any other country in the world.[7] One survey showed that the average office worker is distracted every thirty-one minutes.[8] If you work in the service industry, you're multitasking eleven tasks per shift, and that doubles if you're working the morning shift.[9] The next time the barista gets your morning coffee order wrong, try and show a little compassion instead. They are juggling a large mental load.

Like Holly, you've likely aspired to get better at multitasking or been complimented for your multitasking skills in your professional life. Haven't we all? But multitasking is a scientific misnomer, another long-standing myth our hustle culture likes to perpetuate. When you multitask, what your brain is actually doing is called *task switching*—moving quickly from one task to another in rapid succession. The human brain is wired to do one thing at a time. Studies show that only 2.5 percent of human brains have the uncommon distinction of being able to do more than one thing at a time, but this is exceedingly rare.[10] Most of us are terrible at multitasking, even though 100 percent of us believe we're excellent multitaskers!

Task switching can have a detrimental effect on your brain with respect to cognition, memory, and attention.[11] Studies show that multitasking can slow down your productivity by 40 percent.[12] It makes you less productive because it weakens your prefrontal cortex, the area of your brain responsible for higher executive and cognitive function.[13] Task switching also makes you less skilled at solving complex problems. Our world is filled with complex problems to solve. We can't afford to multitask!

For Holly, that meant another change in perspective: learning to monotask. *Monotasking* is a way to protect your brain from burnout and stress. But you may be thinking "that's how my brain works. I always have three or four things going at once." You might question whether you can maintain your efficiency and accomplish everything expected of you at work and at home if you stop multitasking.

The real-world strategy to efficiently monotask is to create *time blocks*.

For Holly, who often worked on several projects at a time, we devised the following schedule using the Pomodoro Technique.[14] This technique was developed for time management in the late 1980s and has been used with great success by those of us who feel distracted, frazzled, torn in many directions, procrastinate because of overwhelm, or try to keep too many plates spinning at one time. Use a timer and allow yourself twenty-five minutes (called a *pomodoro*—the Italian word for "tomato," which the developer of this technique chose because of the tomato-shaped kitchen timer he used when he was a student) to focus on only one task. You set your timer, and when it rings, you stop and take a five-minute break away from the task. Then, you move on to your second task and put a fresh twenty-five minutes on the timer . . . and repeat. After four pomodoros in a row, you take a longer thirty-minute break.

Holly's time-blocked work session looked like this:

Task 1, twenty-five-minute time block; five-minute break

Task 2, twenty-five-minute time block; five-minute break

Task 3, twenty-five-minute time block; five-minute break

Task 4, twenty-five-minute time block; five-minute break

Longer thirty- to forty-minute break. Then repeat the above sequence.

Using this schedule, Holly agreed to try swapping multitasking for time blocking instead. By the end of the workday, Holly had made progress on all of her competing projects but without her attention being divided among them. She was able to allot dedicated time to each project and immerse herself fully. She allowed her brain to monotask, thereby strengthening her prefrontal cortex, which helped her solve the many complex tech problems she had at work. She was already keeping her phone and other distractions like pop-ups to a minimum, so time blocking and developing her new schedule helped her recover from the multitasking myth and come up for air.

TECHNIQUE #11: Learn the Magic of Monotasking

1. Decide which tasks are a priority for your day.

2. Choose a set amount of time that you believe you're able to focus without your mind wandering. Initially, it might be only ten to fifteen minutes; with practice you may learn to focus for twenty to thirty minutes. Be mindful of your limits and don't overdo it, which may slow your burnout recovery.

3. Pick a task from your list, set a timer, and focus only on the chosen task. Stay true to monotasking until your timer rings.

4. Take a short break and do something physical: stretching, diaphragmatic breathing, walking in the hallway. Maybe drink some water.

5. Reset your timer for another task from your list, then focus on it until the timer rings.

6. Repeat the above through your workday.

7. Congratulate yourself every day for sharpening your focus through monotasking.

Over time, as Holly's burnout improved, she noticed that it became easier for her to enter into a flow state when she was working on interesting projects. The flow state, as mentioned in Chapter 3, is a mind state in which you're fully immersed in an activity and lose track of time. The flow state also has many mental health benefits, including being protective for work-related burnout.[15] "Flow has also been associated with a number of longer-term wellbeing outcomes," says cognitive scientist Richard Huskey. "Everything from buffering against burnout at work to buffering against depression to increasing resilience."[16]

If you've ever been so engrossed in an activity that the time you spent doing it felt like minutes but was actually hours, you've probably experienced the flow state. There are many paths to entering a flow state; some common examples include writing, playing music, creating art, playing sports, dancing, doing DIY projects, and solving puzzles.

Give yourself some grace as you walk yourself back from burnout and come up for air. Start with honoring your breaks, give up your multitasking habit, and adopt monotasking using time blocking instead. With time, maybe you'll find you have the energy to pursue the activities that bring you joy and get you into a state of flow. Holly's journey took more than three months.

As I did with Holly, I encourage you to not rush the process. Your first step in the Fourth Reset is to make sure you give your brain the break it needs to rest and recover before you start chasing flow. Creating a monotasking habit for yourself isn't meant to be another add-on to your growing to-do list. The road to burnout recovery is slow and intentional. Give yourself the time, patience, and self-compassion to get there.

For Holly, as time went on and her monotasking habit became stronger, she was able to do forty-five-minute time blocks with ten-minute breaks. That may be different for you. If you have a high degree of burnout and have been doing your best working with many distractions, you may need to build up to an uninterrupted block of time. Start slow with a ten-minute block of distraction-free time. Set a timer. Keep your phone out of arm's reach, silence your notifications and Slack channels, and dive into your work. When you complete your time block, you can catch up on what you missed. Each week, aim to increase your time block by five minutes until you can comfortably work for twenty-five to thirty consecutive minutes without distractions.

I've used this strategy since medical school and still use it today. My time blocks are now fifty minutes, because I've slowly built up my ability to focus for longer stretches of time, but I started with twenty-five-minute increments suggested by the Pomodoro Technique. In fact, I wrote this book using this time-blocking technique.

When I was a medical student, I didn't know there was something called monotasking. Nor did I know its many brain benefits. But I needed a technique to help me focus on and retain the large amounts of material I was required to learn every week. I stumbled onto a time-blocking technique that worked for me through trial and error and have stayed with it ever since. When you're stressed and under pressure, it feels daunting to take on any task that will take hours to accomplish fully. You can't visualize the totality, but you can imagine getting through twenty to forty-five minutes.

Organizing time into manageable blocks breaks up the task at hand so that it feels more doable. With every time block you finish, you have a sense of completion and a respite. I would feel a rush of relief when my timer rang and I could leave the medical school library to take a walk outside and stretch my legs. Initially, I think I did time blocking for the built-in breaks, because they helped me overcome the mental hurdle of studying vast amounts of material. Now it's become a habit, and I can't work any other way.

Over the years, I've used time blocking with nearly every project

I've been tasked to complete. Sometimes the block is twenty minutes long, sometimes forty-five minutes, but I never go past the fifty-minute mark because psychologically I need that five-to-ten-minute break every hour to reset my brain.

It took me a few decades to master the skill of monotasking. After all, we each have decades of hustle culture to dismantle, and that doesn't happen in an hour, a day, or even weeks. We've all been living the resilience myth without knowing it. Our brains will happily accept our new way to work on a project once we've adapted our schedules to time blocking. Now I can say I wear my monotasking badge as proudly as I once wore my "excellent multitasker" one!

Over several months, Holly shared my enthusiasm and joined the ranks of fully recovered multitaskers. She became a proud monotasker. With these simple and perhaps counterintuitive tweaks to her working style, her productivity flourished.

Your Brain Loves Compartments

One of the reasons that monotasking through time blocking is an effective strategy to combat stress and burnout is because it supports your brain's need for *compartmentalization*.

Nothing made us appreciate our brain's need for compartmentalization more than the pandemic. The majority of us had to work, parent, and live within the same space, day after day. Humans are multidimensional creatures and serve many roles as workers, parents, spouses, friends, and siblings. When you're unnaturally forced to play out each of these roles in the same physical space, it doesn't bode well for your stress and mental health. Talk about a tea kettle of stress! Many of us felt like that kettle of water, with the flame under it being turned from low to high every day. There was no place to let off the steam because we were trapped in our situations.

When you're able to create clear physical delineations for your many roles, you give yourself an opportunity to function well in each of them. You bring different skills and aspects of your personality to the many spheres you inhabit, and being forced to perform to your maximal capacity in each of your roles while under one small roof with others shortchanges your potential to do any of them well. Just like your brain is wired to monotask rather than multitask, you are your most fulfilled, productive, and actualized self when you're not being forced to multipurpose.

Giselle was a mom to a toddler and worked as a medical writer. Her company offered a hybrid work model: work from home or return to the office. Since her husband worked long hours, Giselle did the daily pickup and dropoff of her toddler to and from preschool. This was before and after her one-hour commute each way to her company's office.

"I hated my long commute, so I thought working from home would be a great respite," Giselle explained when she came to see me for worsening stress. "But I'm at my wit's end," she admitted. "I've been totally unproductive. I'm not meeting deadlines and my reputation is suffering. I was known to be the writer who could deliver with a tight deadline. But lately I've been asking for one extension after another."

For Giselle's Rule of 2, her first intervention was to incorporate the Goldilocks Principle into her workday by honoring her breaks. For her second intervention, I suggested the fake commute.

The Fake Commute

Giselle was convinced that her previous long commute to work held no value, but it served two key purposes. Not only did it transport her physically to work, but it also gave her the time to mentally transport herself and prime her brain for work mode. When she gave up her physical daily commute, she lost her ability to gradually transition from home mode to work mode. Instead, within minutes, she was thrust from being a busy mom and wife into focusing on her medical writing from her kitchen table. Giselle's brain needed a commute to transition from wife-mother-homemaker to company employee.

Working from home can have many benefits, so this isn't about advocating that we should all return to the office. Studies show that the length of a commute is inversely correlated with job satisfaction; the shorter your commute, the higher your job satisfaction.[17] Hybrid work has been shown to improve autonomy, productivity, stress, and burnout.[18] In one Gallup Poll, nearly 60 percent of respondents said hybrid work helped decrease their burnout.[19] With these many benefits of hybrid work, it's not surprising that almost 85 percent of workers prefer a hybrid work model than the traditional in-office model.[20] Hybrid work is increasingly becoming the future of work and a new way to reclaim work-life balance.

However, is it possible to reap the benefits of working from home while still maintaining the psychological benefits of a commute to the office? Yes. You can fake your commute.

As Giselle's husband got their son ready for preschool each morning, Giselle got herself dressed and ready for work as if she were going into the office. She set up her workstation at the kitchen table: laptop, water bottle, and a notepad with a quick priority list. She made lunch for her son and then walked with him to preschool. Instead of rushing back home, feeling harried, and starting her day frantically, she started her fake commute. She stopped by a coffee shop and picked up a coffee to go. She walked around the block drinking her coffee and strategizing about her day. When she got to a local park, she sat on a bench for a few minutes to quickly check her calendar on her phone: What meetings did she have scheduled that day? What project was she going to start first? What needed more revisions? What was ready to submit today?

Her fake commute took approximately fifteen minutes, and during those minutes, Giselle was able to transition from home mode into work mode. She felt calm and organized, ready to begin her workday. She entered her home office, which was previously her kitchen table, took a seat, and began working.

When she came in to my office for her follow-up two months later, Giselle was ecstatic. "Every morning, I've been doing my fake commute," she told me. "My productivity is so much better. I've been churning out articles over the past two months. I make sure I take lots of breaks and do something small to manage my stress like we discussed. For the most part, I've been on track and feel great about the changes. This stuff works!"

Through the fake commute and the process of brain compartmentalization, Giselle was feeling engaged and enthusiastic about her work again, without ever returning to the office. Her brain got the breather it needed. Giselle had finally started to feel like she could come up for air.

TECHNIQUE #12: Fake Your Commute

If you work from home or operate a business from your own property, building in buffer time every morning and evening between your work life and your personal life gives you time to reset your brain and your stress.

Establish your time to begin work. Set up your morning so that you get up, get dressed, and are ready to leave the house as if you had a ten-to-fifteen-minute commute to work.

Take those ten to fifteen minutes to leave your personal home life behind and prepare your brain for work. You might take a walk in the neighborhood, pick up coffee nearby, or scan your daily tasks and appointments to map out your workday.

When you return to your home, go straight to your work area as if you have arrived at your job. You're now ready to begin your workday.

At the end of the workday, reverse your fake commute. Leave your work area behind, take a walk, run a quick errand, and begin to transition back to your personal time.

The Power of Rituals

What Giselle was doing well in taking a fake commute every day was establishing a sense of ritual for working from home. "Ritual" used in this context is not associated with any religious tradition—it merely means a pattern you're developing through the psychology of habit.

Rituals are things you do repeatedly and in a certain order. They're a helpful catalyst to prime your brain, helping you create some mental space when you have little to no physical space. When you're forced to multipurpose in one space, a simple ritual can help your brain recognize that a familiar pattern comes next for the role ahead.

Rituals can be powerful change agents for your brain. Psychiatrist Neha Chaudhary says that rituals can help us regulate our emotions. She sees them as "anchors . . . to help us remember who we are and how to navigate life."[21] Sports psychologist Caroline Silby adds, "Rituals allow you to create a pathway to connect your mind and body and feel in control during a time where there are a lot of unknowns . . . [to be] more empowered to respond and make effective choices."[22]

The fake commute can be a potent ritual for change, but you may choose another ritual instead. Aim to take a simple action consistently at the start of your workday that signifies a transition from home mode to work mode. It's less about the actual ritual you decide to use and more about the meaning and purpose you've infused into the action. Some examples of rituals include lighting a candle, turning on a special desk lamp, using a designated coffee mug during work hours, placing your phone in a specific place at least ten feet away from your workstation, using a work-specific pen and notepad, or having a certain set of stretches that you do between each work call. The Stop–Breathe–Be technique would be a great addition to your repertoire of rituals during the workday. Whatever small gestures you choose to use, infuse them with as much intention as possible to send a signal to your brain that you're in work mode. You can also add rituals to times of your workday that are natural starting and stopping points—lunchtime, your coffee break, or the end of the day.

The Bookend Method

Regardless of which ritual you choose, aim to create bookends for your workday, that is, create a definitive declaration to start your workday and another to signal a finite end to it. It can be the same ritual for morning and evening or different ones. But try to make it the same every day so you can habituate your brain to getting out of home mode and into work mode and vice versa. This trains your brain over time to shift gears from one role to another with more ease, freeing up your mental bandwidth to be fully present for whichever role you're inhabiting at that moment.

After the first two months of Giselle perfecting the Goldilocks Principle and the fake commute in the morning, when I saw her in a follow-up visit, we decided to add an evening fake commute to bookend her days. Instead of working until the last possible minute before she was late to pick up her son, Giselle would give herself fifteen minutes to wrap up her tasks. She'd power down her laptop, put it away in her work bag, rinse out her coffee mug, and head outside for her evening fake commute. She'd review what went well that day, what didn't, and which important priorities she needed to tackle the next day. As she walked, she would begin thinking about her son's chubby cheeks and what he'd like to eat for dinner. She also thought about whether she wanted to go to visit her sister over the weekend or wait until the end of the month. When she picked up her son, she was present and joyful. She had come up for air, having fully transitioned out of work mode and back into home mode.

Some of my patients, and this may apply to you as well, can't use the fake commute or bookend method because they don't work at home or at an office job. This was true of Henry, a twenty-four-year-old package delivery driver. His workplace was the company truck, not an office or his home. His high-pressure job required him to drive around the city delivering multiple packages to many addresses.

Henry had to leave college after his first year because his mother became ill and he was her primary caregiver. He married his high school girlfriend and they had a son. His son was now five years old and Henry's pride and joy.

"I would never want to trade being a dad or a husband," Henry said, "but I had to find work right away and didn't get to decide on a career. Now, I drive around all day, worried about what the future holds. You know, how am I ever going to be able to get a decent car, maybe buy a house, and even give my kid and wife a better life? My mind races all day long."

"How do you feel about your job?" I asked.

"Come on, now," Henry said, dropping his head to the side. "Let's face it, I'm not getting anywhere . . . fast. I show up every day, but I always think, is this all I'm ever going to do?"

I could tell that Henry's job dissatisfaction felt like a dead end to him, causing him relentless stress. For the first part of Henry's Rule of 2, I suggested the following technique, which gives your mind a rest no matter what type of work you do.

TECHNIQUE #13: Activate Your Sticky Feet

Each of your feet has almost thirty bones and more than one hundred muscles, tendons, and ligaments. That's a lot of power in one tiny area of your body. Often overlooked, your feet can be a grounding force during chaotic times.

I learned what I call the sticky feet technique when I was doing yoga regularly every week. The teacher would ask us to spread our toes and imagine them being webbed to create more stability during poses. I always loved that imagery. And even though I didn't quite understand what it meant, it did help ground me in the moment on my mat. Soon, I started using it off the mat during other times of the day.

You can practice sticky feet, too. The point is to keep your mind where your feet are. Stand tall and try to imagine your feet as sticky webs, taking up as much surface area as they can. Feel the connection and sturdiness that your feet impart on the ground as they hold you up. Dig in to that support.

You can imagine your sticky feet and *be where your feet are* as you wait for an elevator or pump gas—just about anywhere you're standing upright for a few minutes.

So when you're on the job, practice having sticky feet and *be where your feet are*. When you're home, have sticky feet and *be where your feet are* as you wash dishes at the kitchen sink or brush your teeth in the bathroom. It's always the same catchphrase. No matter where you are physically, stay mentally present *where your feet are*.

This is a main tenet of mindfulness that's difficult to understand in theory but easier to experience in practice. Henry's job of driving from one location to another delivering packages gave him many opportunities throughout the day to practice sticky feet and to be where his feet are—even though he was on the move all day. He could say to himself, in a gentle and compassionate way, *Be where my feet are*. This helped him stay grounded and focused on the task at hand.

Sticky feet is an effective exercise to help you tap into your mind-body connection because it helps to stabilize and ground you using your feet, rather than your breath. Grounding ourselves with our feet first, whether standing still or through mindful movement, helps us stay anchored in the present moment. And having a sense of presence in the here and now is what the mind-body connection is all about.

When you put your focus where your feet are, you minimize the mind-wandering associated with anxiety. Remember, anxiety is a future-focused emotion. Henry's anxiety wasn't about his current package delivery; his angst stemmed from thinking about his future. "What if?" is the question that you ask yourself the most when you're anxious. For Henry, his mental dialogue went something like this: "What if I'm at this job forever? What if I can't find something better? What if I can't make ends meet? What if I can't be the provider I always wanted to be for my family?" And so on. My work with Henry was to help him slow down his what-if thinking and let his brain come up for air.

The what-if train of thought often doesn't come to an end when you're anxious and stressed, it just gains steam. This what-if mentality is driven by your amygdala, your lizard brain, in the same way that your lizard brain drives the train of your maladaptive stress response. Anxiety and stress are so closely tied because they have the same train operator: your amygdala. Going into a spiral of worry about the future is what your amygdala does best.

In Henry's case, I wanted him to focus on being present, wherever his feet happened to be. "When you're delivering one package, be there," I told him. "When you move on to the next package delivery, then be there. We're going to try to sync up your physical state and mental state to minimize your what-if mentality. Notice the neighborhood you're driving in. Look at the trees, the buildings, the curve of the road as you drive. Be where your feet are."

"Okay, but I don't know how that's going to help my worries," Henry said, shrugging.

"You're not giving up. You're giving your biology a break from what-if mode and going into what-is mode. Once your mind is relaxed and present, you'll be able to get more creative about coming up with solutions to your situation."

"What if worries still come in?" Henry asked, then smiled at another what-if question.

"It's normal for you to worry," I said, "but with this technique your worries will have less intensity, with time. And you'll be able to think more clearly when you're less stressed. You can even consider keeping a worry notebook in the van. Write down a couple of words about the worry. Then, you can decide that you don't have to think about it anymore while you're driving."

For Henry's Rule of 2 I also prescribed deep diaphragmatic breathing to help him feel grounded even though he was moving around all day.

Henry sent me an email a month later telling me that these techniques were helping his stress and anxiety. He wanted to give it another month before seeing me in person in my office.

When I saw Henry the following month, he came in and sat down with a big smile on his face. "Okay, let me tell you what happened with your advice," he said. "I started focusing on where my feet are during the day as I delivered packages, and while driving I did my deep breathing exercises. Then, I began taking the packages to the door instead of dropping them on the porch, and if I saw a customer, I'd say 'hi' and talk for a minute or two. I noticed stuff I never have before, like cool-looking trees and funny-looking dogs. I started smiling at other drivers, even if I wasn't feeling it. And most of them smiled back. Even after work, my wife and son were like, 'What's up with you?' because I was happier."

I could feel my eyes starting to tear up. Nothing makes me happier, as a doctor, than to see a patient feel empowered, reset their stress, and feel so much better.

Then Henry jumped to his feet. "But here's the real miracle of it, doc. I deliver to this one sportswear company almost every day. And the other day, the boss-guy at the company came out to the front desk and told me, 'My staff always has nice things to say about their interactions with you. I don't know what your plans are, but I'd like to have you come in and meet with me for a possible position here in my company.'"

I paused and waited, then finally said, "Okay! Spill it! Did you go?"

"Yes ma'am! I start on Monday as a junior resource manager. And I'll be making two times more money than I made at my delivery job!"

I jumped to my feet too, and Henry and I high-fived in midair.

"Being where my feet were ended up solving a lot of my worries," Henry said.

Of course, there's no guarantee of new jobs or solutions to all your concerns by putting your mind where your feet are, but your brain will thank you for it. It also benefits relationships with family and friends. When you're home, or out with a friend, put your mind there, too. Leave your work at your job, as much as possible, and feel more deeply connected with family and friends. Heart health matters, too.

Your life is filled with demands and obligations. Every minute is accounted for, and you're being pulled in many different directions.

Your brain makes it all possible. But it needs rest and recovery to function optimally; it needs to come up for air. The four techniques in this reset—honoring your breaks with the Goldilocks Principle, learning to monotask, creating a fake commute, and activating your sticky feet to keep your mind present where your feet are—can all help support your brain to be the best it can be for you and for everyone else who depends on you.

7

The Fifth Reset: Bring Your Best Self Forward

We each experience stress in a uniquely personal way depending on our individual circumstances. Your canary symptoms are probably very different from someone else's. But one unifying aspect of your stress journey with another's is the appearance of the inner critic during times of stress.

Your inner critic, also known as your *negative self-talk*, is your inner monologue. It's been shaped by your upbringing, personality, experiences, and society. Having lived with your inner critic your whole life, you may not even realize its presence. During periods of low stress, it's barely a whisper. But during periods of unhealthy stress, your inner critic grabs a megaphone. It's the voice in your head that calls you names when you mess up, discourages you from trying something new or difficult, and berates you when things don't go according to plan.

Your inner critic speaks loudly and often during times of unhealthy stress because your inner critic, however misguided, is trying to protect you. As you learned in Chapters 1 and 2, unhealthy stress activates your amygdala. Your self-preservation mechanism goes into overdrive, and your brain functions from a scarcity mindset. Your inner critic is part of your self-preservation machinery.[1]

That's why advice like "just be happy," "think positive," or "try to relax" is utterly unhelpful when you're stressed. Simply thinking stress away doesn't work. If you could do those things, you would have by now.

As you now know, the biology of stress is a runaway train and leaves you scrambling to find the brakes. During my stress story many well-intentioned people in my life, including my doctor, told me to "relax," "look for the positives," and "get over it." In spite of my sincere effort to do all those things, none of them worked. I ended up feeling worse. I was already in a negative headspace with my stress, and my inability to think positive thoughts just added to my scarcity mindset. Thinking yourself out of stress is a fairy tale, and a lot of the advice we get stems from the myth of toxic resilience.

Another reason why your inner critic is particularly loud during periods of unhealthy stress has to do with how stress impacts your sense of self-efficacy. As we explored in Chapter 3, when you achieve your MOST goal, your feelings of self-efficacy go up, which has a therapeutic effect on your well-being. The reason this is so important is because stress weakens your sense of self-efficacy. Unhealthy stress and its many uncomfortable sensations can make you feel out of control. When you're feeling a lack of control, it's easier to start talking to yourself in unkind ways. Your inner critic gets ahold of a megaphone. The voice gets louder, which adds to your feelings of inadequacy and your unhealthy stress. It's a vicious cycle.

The Fifth Reset is about breaking that cycle. It's about taking the megaphone out of your inner critic's grip and reclaiming your power and sense of self-efficacy. Using the two techniques in this reset—

"Catalog Your Gratitude" and "Express Yourself"—you'll learn how to silence your inner critic and bring your best self forward.

Silencing Your Inner Critic

When Robyn came to see me, she was feeling the detrimental effects of her inner critic. She described it as a relentless monologue. Robyn was an entrepreneur with a new company and a new baby. To say she felt overwhelmed by her competing roles was an understatement. Robyn was seeing her therapist and her obstetrician for help and support, and she decided to see me to get some extra guidance after a particularly eventful morning.

"I was late for my first meeting and as I rushed out the door, I spilled the tiniest bit of coffee on my blouse," she told me. "Instead of taking it in stride, I burst into tears and started berating myself, 'I can't do anything right. I'm so incapable. I'm not prepared for this meeting and we're going to lose the deal because of me. I should just stay home.' I was so upset by this tiny coffee stain that I couldn't function all day at work and contemplated going home. The intensity of my negative thoughts over this tiny coffee stain shocked me."

Robyn knew that chronic stress and burnout were causing her unexpected reaction, but she was still perplexed. "I always have a spare blazer in my office that I could've just thrown on to cover the coffee. In hindsight, I went into full doomsday scenario mode. It's just so unusual for me."

Robyn may have been surprised by her out-of-proportion reaction, but I wasn't. It's a common hallmark of the stressed brain to have a heightened sensitivity to negative experiences. Your stressed brain is hypervigilant to the external environment, and even a seemingly insignificant mistake can set off a cascade of negative emotions.

This is yet another manifestation of your amygdala's focus on self-preservation and survival gone haywire.

As psychologist Rick Hanson describes, during stress, negative experiences become sticky in the brain, like Velcro, because that's your brain's way of scanning for danger to keep you safe.[2] This isn't a design flaw in your mental makeup; it's a natural protective mechanism meant to keep you alert and away from harm. It's the same mechanism that compels you to doomscroll social media when you're anxious, like the tribal night watchman who keeps a lookout for danger or invasion while members of the tribe sleep (Chapter 4). Hypervigilance and a heightened sensitivity to negative experiences are hallmarks of any maladaptive stress response.

Robyn needed a short-term solution to tackle her out-of-proportion stress reaction while it happened in real time, but she also needed a long-term strategy to reset her brain out of doomsday mode for good.

For Robyn's Rule of 2, she began with the Stop–Breathe–Be technique (Chapter 5). I asked her to choose two tasks that were part of her morning routine that were particularly triggering for her stress. As a new business owner and first-time mom, Robyn literally hit the ground running at 5:30 a.m. every morning. She didn't need an alarm, as her infant's cry signaled to her that it was time to get up. She would rocket out of bed and into her robe and race down the hallway to the baby's room.

"For some reason, I run like it's an emergency," Robyn told me. "Usually he's cooing at the solar system mobile over his crib when I get there. He's not stressed, so why am I?"

I suggested she apply the Stop–Breathe–Be technique before she stepped inside the baby's room every morning. I wanted her to stop her body completely, ground herself with a deep breath at the doorway to her baby's room, and be fully present and aware in that moment as she responded to her baby's cry. Then, she could go in and pick up her baby.

Robyn sent me an email after her first week: "This little Stop–Breathe–Be trick brings me and my son so much joy each morning. It's setting the tone for my whole day. When I'm at his doorway doing it, he watches me with the biggest smile on his face! I didn't even notice him smiling at me before this. Those three seconds first thing in the morning have made me rethink my entire morning routine."

By practicing the grounding exercise of Stop–Breathe–Be first thing in the morning, Robyn stopped the cascade of stress reactions that followed her early morning sprint to the nursery. When the first moments of her morning were mindful and calm, they created a domino effect and set the tone for the rest of her day.

"I'm using this for so many other parts of my day," she wrote. "I usually scroll through work emails while making coffee, but now I'm doing Stop–Breathe–Be before I get my mug out of the cupboard. And I do it on my way to work after dropping off my son at daycare. It used to be a frantic and rushed time, but things feel different now. I use the technique before I start the ignition. It hardly takes any extra time. It's the reset my brain needs every morning."

Robyn was slowly and purposefully shifting her biology of stress away from survival mode and into a calmer, more grounded state. She was bringing her best self forward. She still had plenty of stress in her life, but beginning her days with Stop–Breathe–Be was having a ripple effect.

In this new state of mind, Robyn felt more in control of her emotions and therefore could afford to use some of her mental bandwidth to think about some long-term solutions to rewire her brain for less stress.

It was time to introduce Robyn to her second intervention for her

Rule of 2, the therapeutic practice of gratitude. Practicing gratitude would help coax her brain out of its doomsday mentality, which is a feature of the scarcity mindset, and back into the abundance mindset.

I knew Robyn wouldn't be particularly open to a gratitude practice, so I explained the science of gratitude and cognitive reframing to her first as a selling point. It worked.

Gratitude: From Velcro to Teflon

The language of gratitude is a powerful circuit breaker for your brain's stress pathway. Gratitude has been shown to decrease stress, improve mood and resilience, and improve life satisfaction.[3] In one study, gratitude was found to be protective for depressive and physical symptoms during a stressful life event; in another, gratitude decreased stress levels in just one month.[4] Gratitude can also help alter your brain circuitry for negative experiences; instead of sticking to you like Velcro, those experiences can slide off like Teflon.[5] This process is known as *cognitive reframing*—that is, what you focus on grows.[6]

"By taking just a few extra seconds to stay with a positive experience . . . you'll help turn a passing mental state into lasting neural structure," says Hanson. "Mental states become neural traits. Day after day, your mind is building your brain."[7]

By teaching your brain the language of gratitude, you're protecting it from some of the harmful effects of stress. By actively cultivating positive thoughts, you're also helping to counteract your inner critic. But let's be clear, gratitude isn't a façade for toxic positivity. This isn't the Pollyanna approach of "everything is fine." You can be struggling with your stress and mental health and still be able to practice gratitude for certain aspects of your life. In one study of three hundred college students gratitude was found to benefit those who were struggling with their stress and mental health.[8]

The researchers described these beneficial changes to mental health as a 'positive snowball effect' that grew with time, "It's important to note that the mental health benefits of gratitude . . . did not emerge immediately, but gradually accrued over time. And this difference in mental health became even larger 12 weeks after the writing activities."[9]

At first, gratitude may feel unnatural to you and may take concentrated effort, especially if your stress pathway has been in overdrive in recent months or years. But as the science shows, gratitude is a practice and a skill to master. But with time and consistency, your brain can learn this new language of gratitude, which can help you silence your inner critic.

When I mentioned starting a gratitude practice to Robyn, she balked. "Gratitude is kind of a hokey thing, right? I'm not a touchy-feely kind of person."

Robyn wasn't enthusiastic about my idea of gratitude as a coping skill, but she agreed to give it a go when I shared the results of a recent study that showed how it could help her burnout. As a new mom and an entrepreneur, Robyn was experiencing two of the most common culprits for burnout and mental health challenges. One study of working parents found that two-thirds of parents, and almost 70 percent of working mothers in particular, met the criteria for burnout.[10] Another study of female entrepreneurs demonstrated that 52 percent experienced mental health conditions and 95 percent experienced anxiety while raising money to build their businesses.[11]

Robyn wasn't the exception; she was the rule. Her symptoms of chronic stress and burnout weren't a personal failing. Instead, they pointed to larger systemic forces like the lack of support for working mothers and female entrepreneurs. Learning these statistics,

Robyn felt emboldened to take the next step on the way to healthy stress that energized her instead of depleting her. She agreed to follow through with gratitude as her second intervention in her Rule of 2.

Robyn started a daily gratitude practice by keeping a notebook and pen on her nightstand so each night before bed she could write down five things she was grateful for that day and why. I had instructed her that this wasn't supposed to be a long writing exercise, but simply something she should do each night for a minute or two.

I told Robyn that her gratitude doesn't have to be about big life-changing thoughts or events. It can be as simple as "I'm grateful to have strong arms to hold my baby" or "I'm grateful there were leftovers so I didn't have to cook tonight."

That's what finally pierced through Robyn's resistance to do it. "Okay," she said, "that seems easy enough."

We also discussed the importance of writing down her list rather than reciting it or even typing it on her phone or her laptop. Our brains use a different neural circuitry when writing by hand as compared with typing. You are more likely to remember something if you write it on paper.[12] Have you ever experienced writing out your grocery list by hand and then forgetting to take it to the store with you? Oddly, you probably remembered almost every item on your list. That most likely wouldn't have happened if you had typed it into your phone and then accidentally deleted it.

Robyn reluctantly started her gratitude practice each night. When she came in to see me four weeks later, her inner critic's monologue of doom and gloom was significantly quieter. "I definitely feel a difference. My frame of mind is less critical of myself and calmer," she told me. "Once in a while, when something happens during the day,

I'll think to myself 'I need to write this down tonight on my gratitude list.' I've also started paying attention to the smaller things now. The word I'd use to describe the change is 'relish.' I'm relishing certain aspects of my life now rather than just moving through the world on autopilot," Robyn said confidently.

Robyn's brain and its pathways had started to shift along with her gradual shift in perspective. She had silenced her inner critic and made space for her best self to come forward instead.

TECHNIQUE #14: Catalog Your Gratitude

1. Place a notebook or pad of paper along with a pen or pencil near your bed.

2. Before you lie down to sleep, write five things in the notebook that you are grateful for. It can be something good that happened during the day or even as simple as having warm water for a shower.

3. Write out a brief statement of why you're grateful for each item on your list.

4. Keep this nightly ritual going for three months and check in with yourself every four weeks to see whether your daily perspective has changed.

During my stress struggle, I also found a daily gratitude practice to be so helpful. Like Robyn, I couldn't imagine what this simple practice would do to improve my level of stress. I was working eighty hours a week, managing illness and death in the hospital wards. I didn't have time, interest, or patience to write about my feelings in a journal like a teenager. I wanted data-driven results. But after surveying the research, I skeptically began my own nightly gratitude practice before bed.

Sometimes it would be a struggle. I'd write things like "I'm grateful for two arms and two legs"; "I'm grateful for a beating heart"; "I'm grateful for lungs that breathe." I had cared for many patients who couldn't say such things, so my gratitude was authentic. If it didn't feel authentic, I didn't write it down. Some days it was hard to come up with five things; other days I wanted to write more than five things. Most nights, in the beginning, I only wanted to turn off the light and try to sleep, but I stayed disciplined and wrote down five things a day. Over time, my thoughts started changing. Like Robyn, I noticed a shift in my perspective from doom and gloom to calm and centered. My inner critic was slowly losing its power. It was an imperceptible change that happened gradually over many weeks.

I distinctly remember walking down the street one sunny, spring Sunday afternoon and having the sudden realization, "Whoa, I haven't heard my inner critic all weekend. In fact, I don't think I've heard it all week!"

It felt like a burden had been lifted off my shoulders. I had learned how to silence my inner critic and bring my best self forward, one gratitude journal entry at a time.

Since that day, I've kept up with my gratitude practice. I don't do it every day like I did in the early years of training my brain for this new language, but whenever life gets stressful, I start consistently writing in my gratitude journal that sits on my nightstand to this day. Without fail, my brain pathways begin to recalibrate away from stress and back toward calm through the process of cognitive reframing. It's now become an invaluable tool in my toolkit during times of stress. I hope it will be the same for you.

Therapeutic Writing

You may begin your gratitude practice reluctantly, like Robyn did, but end up relishing it too. Putting your thoughts and emotions on the page can be a cathartic and therapeutic experience. If you've been through something traumatic, it's even more important to let those painful feelings out. Over the years, many of my patients have released their bottled-up emotions through a scientifically verified writing exercise called *expressive writing*.

Like you, my patients have busy, full, and sometimes chaotic lives. They're held to impossible standards at work and at home. Many of them feel like they're always "on." They don't get the opportunity to let down their guard, which is why many of them have an emotional release the minute the door closes during their office visit with me. It's their opportunity to finally just be. We're human beings, not human doings, and expressive writing can help those of us, who have many forward-facing roles, cope a little better in each of them. And the science supports this.

Expressive writing, developed by social psychologist James Pennebaker, is very straightforward and deceptively simple.[13]

TECHNIQUE #15: Express Yourself

Here are clear instructions on how to practice expressive writing in Pennebaker's own words:[14]

> *I would like you to write about your very deepest thoughts and feeling about an extremely important emotional issue that has affected you and your life. In your writing, I'd like you to really let go and explore your very deepest emotions and thoughts. You might tie your topic to your relationships with others, including parents, lovers, friends, or relatives; to your past, your present,*

or your future; or to who you have been, who you would like to be, or who you are now. You may write about the same general issues or experiences on all days of writing or on different topics each day. All of your writing will be completely confidential. Don't worry about spelling, sentence structure, or grammar. The only rule is that once you begin writing, continue to do so until your time is up.

The effects of expressive writing can be far-reaching. It has been shown to have a positive impact on a wide array of things that influence you and your life, such as physical ailments, depression, emotional distress, your immune system, being rehired after job loss, missed days at work, and if you're a student, your GPA.[15]

One of the most consistent findings from one study to the next on expressive writing is that it decreases the number of your doctor visits because it helps to minimize the physical ailments connected to stress-related disorders, which, as mentioned previously, doctors say factor into 60 percent to 80 percent of patient appointments. Imagine if we could teach patients how to use expressive writing for their stress-related physical symptoms. Then your doctor might be on time for your appointment for once!

I've prescribed expressive writing to many of my patients from every age group and walk of life, and nearly all have gotten some benefit from the exercise. When I was a patient and came out of my own tunnel of stress, I used expressive writing too. I was curious about what had happened to me. Expressive writing uncovered a lot of buried thoughts and feelings about one of the most distressing times of my life. It helped me make sense of and find meaning about that specific moment in time, offering me much-needed perspective and emotional distance. It untangled a lot of my existential knots. I believe that expressive writing is one of the techniques, among the many others outlined in this book, that has helped me never experience that stampede of horses again.

I followed the same writing protocol that Pennebaker studied. I carved out an uninterrupted fifteen to twenty minutes for four consecutive days, set a timer, and started writing. I wrote about the traumatic event of first feeling that stampede of wild horses (see Chapter 1). At the end of my self-experiment, I felt so much better. And you can too.

You don't need to be concerned about anyone else finding or reading your private thoughts. At the end of your writing time, you can shred the paper you've written on and get rid of it. It's not about preserving your emotions; it's about releasing them so they don't boil up into a bigger issue either physically or mentally. It's one more technique for opening the valve on the tea kettle of stress and letting out some therapeutic steam.

If you've been through a challenging and personally traumatic past experience that you believe may be contributing to your current stress, now is the time to process your emotions. Expressive writing helps you drop your emotional baggage so you can travel light on your path toward less stress and more resilience.

Of course, even with techniques that help your biology manage your stress, there are bound to be elements and experiences in life that occasionally sideline you. We all have them. My patient Jeanette (from Chapter 3), the apartment building manager who was recovering from a stroke, came in for a follow-up appointment six months after her first visit. I felt instant concern. She had gained quite a bit of weight and she seemed to have had a setback physically because she was using a cane again.

"Last time I was here, I thought my brain was broken," Jeanette told me. "This time, my heart is broken."

Jeanette filled me in on the details: her partner had left her weeks before they were to go on their cruise. "I was really improving physically," Jeanette said, "but I guess it wasn't quick enough for her. She met someone younger and moved out."

"Jeanette, I'm really sorry that happened," I said. "You must be so sad."

"Sad? I'm damn mad!" Jeanette said, thumping her cane on the floor three times with the same enthusiasm I remembered from our first visit. "She had it good with me. Then, she had the nerve to take our cat with her!"

I felt relief to see Jeanette's spirit, even if it was showing itself as anger.

"The problem is, we have all the same friends," Jeanette said, waving her cane in the air, "so I have no one to talk to about this. I haven't left the apartment in two weeks, except for today."

"I have a new Rule of 2 for you, Jeanette," I said. "First, I want you to make an appointment to see your physical therapist again. Will you do that?"

Jeanette got a twinkle in her eye. "I guess I didn't help my stroke recovery sitting on my butt and eating microwave popcorn and pints of Rocky Road ice cream for lunch and dinner. Okay, I'll go back tomorrow."

Then, I gave her the second Rule of 2, which was expressive writing. I explained the technique to her and printed out Pennebaker's description to take with her.

A month later, I checked in on Jeanette by phone. "I'm in a condo on the Jersey shore!" she told me with excitement in her voice. "My big-shot cousin bought a bunch of them and needed somebody to keep an eye out and report to him if anybody needed repairs or anything."

"What a great change, Jeanette!" I said.

"After I left your office, I did that expressive writing for the next week. Boy, did I let some stuff out about my ex! I had to rip it up and toss it all down the garbage chute in the apartment building," she said. "I'll tell you what, though, it worked! I still have moments of anger and sadness, especially about the cat and not getting to take that cruise. But now I've got a whole beach! So I can't complain."

When I asked her how she was doing physically, she replied, "It's been a slow go, but hey, the cane is in the closet and I walk the boardwalk every day. I have salads for lunch and I've lost three pounds."

Before I hung up, I asked whether her broken heart was mending, too. Jeanette paused and then said, "You know, I look out at the ocean from my balcony and I think about how the tide goes out but it always comes back in before too long. Right? I guess life is like that, too."

I knew Jeanette would be better than fine. She was now experiencing healthy stress, and her true resilience was shining through to my Boston office all the way from the Jersey shore. She had found a way to bring her best self forward.

When I prescribed this technique to Carmen (from Chapter 3), the lawyer-turned-artist, at her follow-up, I didn't know that it would be her last Rule of 2. Her experimental cancer therapy hadn't worked, and her ovarian cancer had spread to her liver. Yet she was calm and smiling.

"Now what?" Carmen asked rhetorically. "Am I just supposed to give up, curl into a ball, and die? I'm not ready. I have things to do."

In spite of looking a little more frail, Carmen was beaming with pride when she gave me an invitation to her gallery show in three weeks.

Since our previous visit, Carmen had made great progress cultivating her eudaimonic happiness. Her Rule of 2 had helped her find meaning and purpose in her sculptures and by spending time in nature.

"There's just one thing I can't shake," she said. "I distinctly remember the day I got my promotion when I was working as a lawyer. I didn't want to accept it. I hated my job. But my colleague convinced me to take it, so I did. I regret going against my better judgment. Who knows what could've happened in my life if I had said 'no' like my inner voice told me to."

Carmen still had some unfinished business. To validate and normalize her difficult experience and to help her feel less isolated in her regret, I shared with her some compelling research. The most common regret people have at the end of their life is, *I wish I'd had the courage to live a life true to myself, not the life others expected of me.*[16]

Carmen couldn't go back and make a different choice; none of us can. But she could do the next best thing: she could write about it. So I prescribed the expressive writing exercise. Carmen spent twenty uninterrupted minutes over four consecutive days writing about her pent-up anger, rage, self-doubt, and regret.

Live a Lifetime in a Day

I had one final suggestion for Carmen, one that I find to be helpful no matter your age, culture, economic status, employment, or state of physical health, whether you think you have seventy years in front of you, or seventy days. It's a reframe I've often repeated to patients: *Live a lifetime in a day.*

My role in patients' care is to help them uncover their innate resilience, optimism, and well-being. Whether the patient sitting before me is facing the complexities of terminal cancer, chronic pain, or the slings and arrows of life in general, learning to live a lifetime in a day is one of the most universally applicable principles I recommend.

Living a lifetime in a day isn't the maxed-out approach to a twenty-four-hour period you may be imagining. It's the antidote to hustle culture. It's about slowing down. Living a lifetime in a day is about incorporating the six elements that make up an arc of a long and meaningful life—childhood, work, vacation, community, solitude, and retirement—and building each of those into *one single day*. By practicing how to live a lifetime in a day, you can gradually redefine your sense of time, which is your most cherished and endangered currency, in a new and welcoming way. Living a lifetime in a day can gift you with a rich sense of satisfaction at the end of each day. Because we are all on borrowed time after all.

Here are the six elements to living a lifetime in a day. These elements aren't simply nice-to-haves, they make sound clinical and psychological sense. Allow yourself to incorporate each of these six stages of life into one single day.

- *Childhood*: Spend some of your day in childhood, especially if you're an adult. Cultivate your sense of wonder and play. Create joy for joy's sake. Find your flow state, which we explored in Chapter 3 as the optimal form of happiness.

- *Work*: Take some time every day to work, whether paid or unpaid. This is your opportunity to foster your sense of productivity and achievement, since studies confirm that work of many kinds has the ability to create engagement, purpose, and meaning in our lives, particularly as we age.[17]

- *Vacation*: Take a vacation every day, to unplug, relax, and escape. This is all about pleasure. Focus on what brings you contentment: reading, baking, making art, playing music, swimming, or even watching your favorite show on Netflix. It's about taking a mental holiday.

- *Community*: Spend time every day with your family or community. Connect with people who give you a sense of belonging—friends who feel like family, close colleagues, neighbors. It doesn't have to be a prolonged amount of time, even a quick call can foster connection. Numerous studies have shown us that human relationships are the single most important predictor of happiness in our lifetimes.[18]

- *Solitude*: It's also important to spend some time in solitude every day. Solitude can increase feelings of well-being and can also help spark creativity and our natural ability to respond well to others.[19]

- *Retirement*: And finally, consider some time in retirement each day as a moment to pause, reflect, and take stock of your activity and achievements, both big and small. Paradoxically, the older we are, the happier we become.[20]

These six elements of living a lifetime in a day are applicable to virtually everyone. When I've suggested it to my terminally ill patients who may have only weeks or months to live, it's given them vitality so they can live out their remaining days feeling strong and significant. For my chronically ill patients, it's allowed them to feel momentum and progress, even during moments when their illness becomes debilitating. For my otherwise healthy but stressed patients, it's realigned their focus as they engage more fully in their lives.

Regardless of where you find yourself in your life, living a lifetime in a day can help you stay mindful and present as you move through your day no matter the circumstance you're currently facing. It's a panoramic lens that helps you take the long view of life, and by design, it lets you bring your best self forward.

A Love Letter to Yourself

As you've learned in this Fifth Reset, words and imagery can be powerful tools to help you bring your best self forward during periods of maladaptive stress. That's because humans are primarily visual learners, so most of us learn best when we have visual cues to rely on. As you embark on your journey to less stress, consider using that information to your benefit. Try incorporating visual cues and messages of self-love into your everyday life to help you move forward.

Display your MOST goal and the Backwards Plan to get there in plain sight on your fridge, so it's easy to see every day. Create a daily reminder in your calendar for your walk or gratitude practice. Put up a weekly checklist with your Rule of 2 where you can see it; when you make it through each day, add a big checkmark and spend a few seconds basking in your sense of accomplishment. Use as many visual reminders as you need to remind yourself that you are stronger than your stress. And each morning, make a choice to choose yourself over your stress.

During my own stress story, I used many visual cues to keep me focused on my future self. I wrote down inspirational quotes or messages of encouragement to myself on Post-Its and placed them around my studio apartment. One of my favorites was, "You are allowed to be both a masterpiece and a work in progress, simultaneously."[23] It helped me find more compassion toward myself during my stress story. I also made a large poster to prop up in my apartment's entrance. It simply said *DO* in large black-and-white lettering. Nothing else. As I would come and go, my eyes would naturally fall on that bold print, and it would help propel me into action. I needed that reminder often. You don't need an app, Smartwatch, or other high-tech reminders. A marker and a piece of cardboard work just as well.

A month after our last visit together, Carmen sent me this email: "Thank you, Dr. Nerurkar. I followed your advice with the writing and sculpture and nature. I put a piece of posterboard in my bedroom that says, 'Live a Lifetime in Every Day,' and I've been doing that. I never knew the difference between being healed and being cured, but now I do. I'll never be cured, but at least I finally feel healed."

I saved that email.

Carmen had her gallery show a few weeks later surrounded by her family, friends, and former colleagues in attendance. Her sister sent me photos from the show of Carmen looking radiant and joyful, a picture of deep fulfillment.

Carmen died two months later.

Carmen's end of life had been infused with joy, meaning, purpose, and fulfillment. While never cured, Carmen finally felt healed. She had wholeheartedly embraced the techniques in the Fifth Reset—writing out her gratitude and experimenting with therapeutic writing—along with the principles of living a lifetime in a day. Through coping with her unimaginable illness experience, Carmen had found her way to bring her best self forward. Along the way, she helped so many of us who cared for her become better versions of ourselves. I often think of our enlightening conversations. Carmen may have started off as a student of stress, but watching her come to terms with the end of her life it was clear: the student had become the teacher.

8

The Fast Track

> And then the day came when the risk to remain tight in a bud was more painful than the risk it took to blossom.
>
> —ATTRIBUTED TO ANAÏS NIN

You now have the full scope of all The 5 Resets and fifteen techniques that were each designed to help you overcome your unhealthy, maladaptive stress. We've walked together this far, but the last part of your journey you'll take alone. It's time to bring into your life as action the knowledge you've learned on the page, using the techniques of The 5 Resets and the Resilience Rule of 2 as tools in your toolkit. It's now up to you to pick up the tools and put them to good use, because the resets and techniques only work when you do.

It may feel daunting, and we've discussed the many reasons why change is scary, but I know you're ready, and somewhere deep down you know this too. Even if you're not fully confident in your ability to make change happen, take the first step anyway. I'm cheering you on from a distance. Besides, I have the utmost confidence in your ability to do this for yourself. So consider this my official invitation: it's your moment to begin the brave and rewarding process of bringing change into your life!

How Your Brain Makes Change Happen

I can't believe I let things get this bad before I decided to make a change. I've heard this countless times from my patients, as well as my friends and family. I've even said it to myself. Having this thought isn't a sign that you're failing; it's a sign of progress. From a scientific point of view, having this realization or something similar is the natural pathway toward change that your brain needs to take. So when you say this yourself, know that you are much closer to making change happen than you think!

Even though our hustle culture tells us stories about people who've had one inspirational, life-altering moment that propelled them to make a 180-degree turn, that's fiction and not reality. I've never had a patient tell me that only one moment in time got them to change. Change isn't a one-time event. It's a thousand pivotal moments building momentum and gaining steam over time. Change is a slow dawning, often born out of being fed up with how things are.

Researchers working with smokers in the late 1970s developed what they called the Stages of Change Model, or the Transtheoretical Model of change, identifying five stages:[1]

1. *Precontemplation*: You may or may not be aware of the warnings of your canary and you certainly haven't recognized that it's a problem for you yet. In fact, you may even defend against those warnings.

2. *Contemplation*: You're gradually realizing that those canary warnings may be a problem for you, but you're still not ready for

change. You're weighing your options, wondering whether it's better to ignore the warnings rather than do something about them.

3. *Preparation*: You've decided you want to do something about your canary's warnings. For instance, you're reading this book and figuring out which of The 5 Resets you can bring into your life.

4. *Action*: You're finally ready to act to take care of those warnings. You put The 5 Resets into practice, two techniques at a time (your Rule of 2), and begin to reap the benefits of less stress and more resilience.

5. *Maintenance*: Through a small amount of sustainable effort, you've brought The 5 Resets into your everyday life. Your brain has created new pathways for less stress and more resilience and is being wired differently through your action.

If you think back to some of the biggest changes you've made in your life, like changing jobs or starting a new relationship, you most likely went through these five stages of change before making the final decision to act. So if you're feeling down and wondering to yourself, *How did I let things get so bad?,* show yourself some compassion instead and congratulate yourself. You're probably in the second or third stage of making change happen, much farther along the path than you think.

Trust the Process

These five stages that your brain and body go through before you make the decision to act can happen a little differently for each person. Your healing journey will be unique to you. So if you've felt anxious, angry, frustrated, disappointed, fearful, or even sometimes indifferent as you go through these stages of your stress journey, recognize that every emotion you experience is valid and normal. Growth is a messy, nonlinear process. The trick is to trust the process and keep going, even through the messy middle. Some days you'll take big leaps, and other days you'll feel like you've barely made a dent. But no matter your trajectory or speed, trust that you're making progress on your stress journey. Because you are.

As you bring the techniques offered in The 5 Resets into your life, two at a time, you may sometimes get frustrated that you're not changing fast enough. We all want the fast track to less stress and more resilience. It's so tempting to skip the in-between steps and get to the finish line. Of course it is, because our hustle culture values speed as a modern virtue. But your brain and body have their own timelines. They work at their own, unhurried pace. The mindset shifts, practices, and techniques laid out in this book honor that timeline. To change your biology, you need to work with the timeline of your biology rather than compete against it. Taking slow, small, and steady steps is the surest, most sustainable, and long-lasting path to your finish line of less stress and more resilience.

Remember the children's story "The Hare and the Tortoise"? Your brain and body are a lot like that when it comes to making progress with your stress:

A Hare was making fun of the Tortoise one day for being so slow.

"Do you ever get anywhere?" he asked with a mocking laugh.

"Yes," replied the Tortoise, "and I get there sooner than you think. I'll run you a race and prove it."

The Hare was much amused at the idea of running a race with the Tortoise, but for the fun of the thing he agreed. So the

Fox, who had consented to act as judge, marked the distance and started the runners off.

The Hare was soon far out of sight, and to make the Tortoise feel very deeply how ridiculous it was for him to try a race with a Hare, he lay down beside the course to take a nap until the Tortoise should catch up.

The Tortoise meanwhile kept going slowly but steadily, and, after a time, passed the place where the Hare was sleeping. But the Hare slept on very peacefully; and when at last he did wake up, the Tortoise was near the goal. The Hare now ran his swiftest, but he could not overtake the Tortoise in time.

The race is not always to the swift.[2]

Imagine if the tortoise started second-guessing his abilities during the race: "I'm so slow. I'll never win this race. The hare is so much faster than me. I'm going to get crushed. Why bother trying? I'm going to fail anyway. I might as well give up. Forget this crap. I'm done."

No doubt, the tortoise's negative self-talk would've sabotaged his efforts.

But that's not what happened. The tortoise didn't buy into the hype of speed. He trusted that his slow-moving, steadfast nature would win out in the end. He was unfazed by his pace and instead focused on his tenacity and perseverance.

Have the tortoise mindset. Focus on taking two small steps forward at a time. Start low and go slow. Maybe your two steps will be deciding to walk around the block every day and spending one of your breaks at work doing some gentle stretches rather than scrolling through social media. Whatever your two steps, keep them small and focused. Over time, you'll gradually be ready to take two more steps because you made the first two easy and manageable to bring into your life.

Some days will be easier than others. On the days that feel

impossible, at the very least, ask yourself: *What's the one thing I can do for five minutes that will make me feel better today?* Even if you can do only five minutes of diaphragmatic breathing on a certain day, you are still sending the message to your brain and your body that you are resetting your stress. On days you can't put any energy or time into resetting your stress, give yourself some grace and start again the next day. Research shows that occasional missed opportunities don't negatively affect your brain's ability to form healthy habits for less stress.[3] Hiccups are part of the process of change. Keep moving forward whenever you can.

As you apply The 5 Resets to your life, think about how supportive you would be of someone you love, how you would cheer on their determination and forgive them their missteps, how you would try to have compassion and understanding for what they are going through. Then, apply that same treatment to yourself. Because every step forward counts.

Be Gentle with Yourself

Compassion for yourself when you're feeling stressed isn't an easy emotion to cultivate in the moment, but it can have a profound effect on your stress. Trying to be a little more compassionate with yourself on your stress journey can be one of the most effective paths forward. Nearly all of the techniques in The 5 Resets work more efficiently when you're able to view yourself through the lens of self-compassion. That's because compassion can help change your brain and body, acting as a protective buffer against your stress.

Research shows that self-compassion can decrease cortisol levels, help you cope with difficult life events, and protect your mental health, thereby helping to improve your stress.[4] Compassion can also act on specific brain regions that govern stress like your amygdala.

One study examined brain scans in forty people and found that the amygdala was more active when people were being self-critical and less active when people practiced compassionate self-reassurance.[5] In another study of forty-six women, those with higher levels of self-compassion were found to have lower levels of perceived stress.[6] But it's so much easier to be self-critical, rather than self-compassionate, when you're stressed. Why is it that we're our own worst critic at a time when we'd be better off being our biggest cheerleader?

"We are deeply attached to our self-criticism, and at some level we probably think that pain is helpful," write Kristin Neff and Chris Germer, two psychologists who study self-compassion. "You might say that the motivation of self-compassion arises from love, while the motivation of self-criticism arises from fear."[7]

For so many of my patients, stress and fear have often gone hand in hand. Your brain processes fear and stress in the same region, your amygdala, so that makes sense. But with the lens of self-compassion, you can reframe your fear and stress, through the techniques offered in The 5 Resets, to a brighter future for your mental health. The good news is that self-compassion, along with everything else in this book, is a skill that can be learned, practiced, and perfected thanks to your brain's incredible ability of neuroplasticity.

According to Neff and Germer, "If we truly care about ourselves, we will do things that will help ourselves be happy, such as taking on challenging new projects or learning new skills."[8]

Taking on challenges and learning new skills is what The 5 Resets is all about.

Choose Your Future Self

I've witnessed firsthand hundreds of patient transformations through my clinical practice and heard the success stories from people who attended my talks. Many of these people were on the fast track to burnout and chronic health issues, and some even permanently damaged their relationships and their jobs because of how they handled their stress. You wouldn't have bet on them to succeed in their stress struggle because they had everything going against them, but they made it through their dark tunnel of stress to share their success story with me.

I've asked many of these people—whose biology is identical to yours and mine—how they became their own success story. What did they think, believe, and ultimately do to crawl out from under their specter of stress? Each one of them told me the same thing in their own words. If there was one common thread linking all of these stories, it's that their will to want something better for themselves finally overtook their need to stay the same. *They chose their future self.*

Imagine living your life as your future self with less stress. Envision your future self succeeding and achieving your MOST goal. How would you behave? What actions would you take every day? What would you tell yourself on your way to success? It's easy to get in your own way when it comes to staying the course of any health journey. But if you can see it, you can be it. Visualizing yourself as already successful can help you stay the course and keep the momentum going of The 5 Resets, even when things get challenging on your stress journey. Think of yourself as a success story in the making, and your brain will help you get there one reset at a time. As author Brené Brown has said, "One day you will tell your story of how you overcame what you went through, and it will be someone else's survival guide."

Trust in your ability to be resilient. It's on its way.

Progress Not Perfection

As you move closer to your future self, step by step, you may lose sight of where you started and how far you've come on your stress journey. We are inaccurate historians when it comes to our own progress. When you're living it day after day, it's hard to see the distance you've traveled. If you've ever been on a fitness or weight-loss journey, you know what I mean. You don't really think you're making any day-to-day progress. The people in your life—family, roommates, colleagues—don't notice any changes. But then you go on a weekend away with a friend you haven't seen in six months, and she can't get over how different you look. That's why using something objective to measure your progress is so important.

At the start of this book, you completed a few exercises like figuring your baseline Personalized Stress Score, creating your MOST goal, and designing a Backwards Plan approach to help you achieve it. These are all excellent, objective metrics you can use to track your progress. While you're bringing The 5 Resets into your life, check in with yourself every four weeks and ask yourself these questions:

- What's my new Personalized Stress Score?
- Does my original MOST goal still feel like the right goal?
- Does another MOST goal fit better with where I am currently?
- What step am I currently on in my Backwards Plan?
- Are my current Rule of 2 techniques now wired in my brain?
- Can I add two more techniques to get closer to my future self and MOST goal?

You may not think much has changed with your stress, but when you check in with yourself at four weeks, again at eight weeks, and then at twelve weeks, you'll be amazed at how much progress you've made and how far you've truly come.

It's also important to recognize that growth can be happening internally, even if you can't visibly see it from the outside. One of my favorite examples of growth comes from the natural world, specifically the Chinese bamboo tree, which doesn't show any signs of growth for the first five years but then it grows as much as ninety feet in six weeks! The wonder of this natural phenomenon is the incredible amount of internal change that happens in the first five years that's simply invisible to the outside world. Ninety feet in six weeks may seem sudden, but it isn't: small, incremental changes have to happen internally before the big, visible changes can occur for everyone to see. Of course, it's not going to take you five years to see changes in your stress, but the bamboo is a good reminder that growth can be happening on the inside even if you can't see it on the outside.

When I was early in my stress struggle, I found comfort in a concept Jon Kabat-Zinn in one of his recordings: *Cultivating a new practice within ourselves is like growing a garden. When you plant seeds in a garden, you give them time to sprout into saplings. You treat the tender saplings with gentleness and compassion.*[9] Try to view the techniques of The 5 Resets that you're bringing into your life in the same way. Give them time to grow strong roots and sprout.

On your journey, focus on your progress—forget perfection. It's a myth that doesn't exist. It's easy to get so wrapped up in the final destination, your MOST goal, that you lose sight of the tremendous and valuable work you're doing along the way. You'll eventually get to that goal you've set for yourself, but every step you take on your journey is one step closer to improving your stress.

When you realize you've made progress, celebrate every single win, both big and small. The big wins are easy to celebrate because they're easy to see, but the small ones that you've worked equally hard for are just as important to honor. Congratulate yourself on moving forward and keep going!

The Perfect Storm and the Raincoat

Over the years, I've been honored to witness the transformations of many of my patients who stepped into future selves. My favorite moment of each of their stories is the light bulb moment. It's that moment when you can literally see a flicker of hope and understanding in someone's eyes. My patients will say to me, "Dr. Nerurkar, you fixed my stress!" My response is always the same: "No, I didn't fix your stress. YOU fixed your stress! I was just a mirror." It's my highest belief that you have the power within you to heal your own stress. I simply serve as a mirror on your journey to reflect back all of your progress. I can give you the tools, instructions, and data, but only you can reset your own stress.

That work is in your hands. And so is my belief in you.

The techniques in this book are meant to gradually change your brain and body for less stress in the now, but they're also meant to protect you from stress in the future. Inevitably, you're going to be faced with unexpected and challenging storms in your life. I hope these techniques can serve as your raincoat, to keep you warm, safe, and dry to weather any perfect storm.

During your stormiest days, I want you to remember these words by Pema Chödrön:

> "You are the sky. Everything else—it's just the weather."

Acknowledgments

There are many people who've helped to bring the ideas in *The 5 Resets* from my writing desk and into your hands. My literary agent at WME, Mel Berger, a legend among literary agents who encouraged me for nearly a decade as I contemplated writing this book. My editor Anna Paustenbach at HarperOne, who guided me through every stage of book creation with kindness and compassion. The many dedicated people at HarperCollins Publishers, HarperOne, and WME who gave *The 5 Resets* their care and attention—Judith Curr, Laina Alder, Aly Mostel, Chantal Tom, Jessie Dolch, Melinda Mullin, Ann Edwards, Ty Anania, and many others. Marcia Wilkie, my writing partner and "book therapist," who helped me to humanize the science and kept me buoyant during the writing process. Lori Lousararian and Tracy Cole, at Rogers and Cowan PMK, who amplified the reach of *The 5 Resets* and its message. My speaking agent, Jennifer Bowen, and the entire Leigh Bureau team, for championing my work to audiences around the world. My mentors and collaborators at Harvard Medical School, Beth Israel Deaconess Medical Center and Cooper University Hospital—Russ Phillips, Nancy Oriol, Gloria Yeh, Ted Kaptchuk, Roger Davis, Kelly Orlando, Jayne Sheehan, Jill and Hung Cheng, Vijay Rajput, Anna Headley and Ed Viner—who taught me about doctoring and humanism in medicine. My patients, who were an honor to care for and who taught me so much in return.

My media powerhouse friends—Arianna Huffington, Eve Rodsky, Sweta Chakraborty, and Laurie Siedman—who've encouraged me to be fearless and play big. My inner circle—Kristin Hurst, Arati Karnik, Chrissa Santoro, Shuma Panse, Berett Shaps, Natalie Meyer, Rachel Daricek, Jyoti Phadke, Debra and Doug Williams, and Beth and Marty Magid—whose steadfast friendship has helped to turn my dreams into reality. My parents, Anil and Meena Nerurkar, who've given me everything and taught me to live with enthusiasm and purpose. My wonderful extended family—the Nerurkars, the Vazes, and the Graysons—in the US, India, and the Netherlands—for my sense of tribe and lots of laughter. And most importantly, Mac and Zoe, the two greatest blessings in my life. Everything I do is more joyous and meaningful because I get to share it with you.

Notes

INTRODUCTION

1. Oracle and Workplace Intelligence, LLC, "AI@Work Study 2020: As Uncertainty Remains, Anxiety and Stress Reach a Tipping Point at Work," 2020, https://www.oracle.com/a/ocom/docs/oracle-hcm-ai-at-work.pdf.
2. "Burnout Nation: How 2020 Reshaped Employees' Relationship to Work," Spring Health, December 2020, https://springhealth.com/wp-content/uploads/2020/12/Spring-Health-Burnout-Nation.pdf.

CHAPTER ONE: WHAT'S YOUR STRESS REALLY TELLING YOU?

1. Aditi Nerurkar, Asaf Bitton, Roger B. Davis et al., "When Physicians Counsel About Stress: Results of a National Study," *JAMA Internal Medicine* 173, no. 1 (2013): 76–77, https://doi.org/10.1001/2013.jamainternmed.480.
2. J. Porter, C. Boyd, M. R. Skandari et al., "Revisiting the Time Needed to Provide Adult Primary Care," *Journal of General Internal Medicine* 38 (2023): 147–55, https://doi.org/10.1007/s11606-022-07707-x.
3. US Preventive Services Task Force, "U.S. Preventive Services Task Force Issues Draft Recommendation Statements on Screening for Anxiety, Depression, and Suicide Risk in Adults," USPSTF Bulletin, September 20, 2022, https://www.uspreventiveservicestaskforce.org/uspstf/sites/default/files/file/supporting_documents/depression-suicide-risk-anxiety-adults-screening-draft-rec-bulletin.pdf.
4. Brian Walker and David Salt, "The Science of Resilience," Resilience.org, November 27, 2018, https://www.resilience.org/the-science-of-resilience/.
5. Dike Drummond, "Are Physicians the Canary in the Coal Mine of Medicine?," *You Can Be a Happy MD*, January 21, 2013, https://www.thehappymd.com/blog/bid/285686/are-physicians-the-canary-in-the-coal-mine-of-medicine.
6. Sheldon Cohen, Tom Kamarck, and Robin Mermelstein, "A Global Measure of Perceived Stress," *Journal of Health and Social Behavior* 24, no. 4 (December 1983): 385–96, https://doi.org/10.2307/2136404.

7. "Workplace Burnout Survey: Burnout Without Borders," Deloitte.com, accessed October 4, 2014, https://www2.deloitte.com/us/en/pages/about-deloitte/articles/burnout-survey.html.
8. "The World Health Report 2001: Mental Disorders Affect One in Four People," World Health Organization, September 28, 2001, https://www.who.int/news/item/28-09-2001-the-world-health-report-2001-mental-disorders-affect-one-in-four-people.
9. "Burn-out an 'Occupational Phenomenon': International Classification of Diseases," World Health Organization, May 28, 2019, https://www.who.int/news/item/28-05-2019-burn-out-an-occupational-phenomenon-international-classification-of-diseases.
10. "Stress in America: Money, Inflation, War Pile on to Nation Stuck in COVID-19 Survival Mode," American Psychological Association, March 10, 2022, https://www.apa.org/news/press/releases/stress/2022/march-2022-survival-mode.
11. "Mental Health Replaces COVID as the Top Health Concern Among Americans," Ipsos, September 26, 2022, https://www.ipsos.com/en-us/news-polls/mental-health-top-healthcare-concern-us-global-survey.
12. "Asana Anatomy of Work Index 2022: Work About Work Hampering Organizational Agility," Asana, April 5, 2022, https://investors.asana.com/news/news-details/2022/Asana-Anatomy-of-Work-Index-2022-Work-About-Work-Hampering-Organizational-Agility/default.aspx.
13. Jean M. Twenge and Thomas E. Joiner, "Mental Distress Among U.S. Adults During the COVID-19 Pandemic," *Journal of Clinical Psychology* 76, no. 12 (December 2020): 2170–82, https://pubmed.ncbi.nlm.nih.gov/33037608/; Anjel Vahratian, Stephen J. Blumber, Emily P. Terlizzi, and Jeannine S. Schiller, "Symptoms of Anxiety or Depressive Disorder and Use of Mental Health Care Among Adults During the COVID-19 Pandemic—United States, August 2020–February 2021," *Morbidity and Mortality Weekly Report* 70, no. 13 (April 2021): 490–94, https://www.ncbi.nlm.nih.gov/pmc/articles/PMC8022876/.
14. Joe Gramigna, "Adults' Unmet Mental Health Care Need Has Increased Since Onset of COVID-19 Pandemic," Helio Psychiatry, April 1, 2021, https://www.healio.com/news/psychiatry/20210401/adults-unmet-mental-health-care-need-has-increased-since-onset-of-covid19-pandemic; Anjel Vahratian, Emily P. Terlizzi, Maria A. Villarroel et al., "Mental Health in the United States: New Estimates from the National Center for Health Statistics," September 23, 2020, https://www.cdc.gov/nchs/data/events/nhis-mental-health-webinar-2020-508.pdf.
15. "Pandemic Parenting: Examining the Epidemic of Working Parental Burnout and Strategies to Help," Office of the Chief Wellness Officer and College of Nursing, The Ohio State University, May 2022, https://wellness.osu.edu/sites/default/files/documents/2022/05/OCWO_ParentalBurnout_3674200_Report_FINAL.pdf.
16. Kristy Threlkeld, "Employee Burnout Report: COVID-19's Impact and 3

Strategies to Curb It," Indeed.com, March 11, 2021, https://www.indeed.com/lead/preventing-employee-burnout-report.

17. Aditi Nerurkar, Asaf Bitton, Roger B. Davis et al., "When Physicians Counsel About Stress: Results of a National Study," *JAMA Internal Medicine* 173, no. 1 (2013): 76–77, https://jamanetwork.com/journals/jamainternalmedicine/fullarticle/1392494.

CHAPTER TWO: WHAT YOUR BRAIN THINKS ABOUT STRESS

1. Aditi Nerurkar, "The Trauma of War on Ukrainian Refugees," Forbes.com, March 4, 2022, https://www.forbes.com/sites/aditinerurkar/2022/03/04/the-psychology-of-the-refugee-experience-ukraine/?sh=52a42b9668dd.
2. Bill Hathaway, "Yale Researchers Find Where Stress Lives," YaleNews, May 27, 2020, https://news.yale.edu/2020/05/27/yale-researchers-find-where-stress-lives; Elizabeth V. Goldfarb, Monica D. Rosenberg, Dongju Seo, R. Todd Constable, and Rajita Sinha, "Hippocampal Seed Connectome-Based Modeling Predicts the Feeling of Stress," *Nature Communications* 11 (2020): 2650, https://www.nature.com/articles/s41467-020-16492-2.
3. Aditi Nerurkar, "Meditation vs. Medication: Which Should You Choose?," HuffPost.com, last updated July 30, 2013, https://www.huffpost.com/entry/benefits-of-meditation_b_820177.
4. Thomas H. Holmes and Richard H. Rahe, "The Social Readjustment Rating Scale," *Journal of Psychosomatic Research* 11, no. 2 (August 1967): 213–18, https://www.sciencedirect.com/science/article/abs/pii/0022399967900104?via%3Dihub.
5. Peter A. Noone, "The Holmes–Rahe Stress Inventory," *Occupational Medicine* 67, no. 7 (October 2017): 581–82, https://academic.oup.com/occmed/article/67/7/581/4430935.
6. Gretchen Rubin, "What You Do Every Day Matters More Than What You Do Once in a While," *The Happiness Project*, November 7, 2011, https://gretchenrubin.com/articles/what-you-do-every-day-matters-more-than-what-you-do-once-in-a-while/.

CHAPTER THREE: THE FIRST RESET

1. The originator of this model is unknown though many similar models appear across the internet. See, for instance, Robby Berman, "Who Do You Want to Be During COVID-19?: One Woman's Viral Roadmap from Fear to Learning to Growth," BigThink.com, April 30, 2020, https://bigthink.com/health/covid-graphic-growth-zones/.
2. Jon Kabat-Zinn, *Full Catastrophe Living: Using the Wisdom of Your Body and Mind to Face Stress, Pain, and Illness* (New York: Bantam, 2013), xlix.
3. Thomas Oppong, "The Only Time You Are Actually Growing Is When You're Uncomfortable," CNBC.com, August 13, 2017, https://www.cnbc.com/2017/08/11/the-only-time-you-are-actually-growing-is-when-youre-uncomfortable.html.

4. Kaitlin Woolley and Ayelet Fishbach, "Motivating Personal Growth by Seeking Discomfort," *Psychological Science* 33, no. 4 (2022): 510–23, https://journals.sagepub.com/doi/10.1177/09567976211044685; Kira M. Newman, "Embracing Discomfort Can Help You Grow," *Greater Good Magazine*, May 3, 2022, https://greatergood.berkeley.edu/article/item/embracing_discomfort_can_help_you_grow.
5. Laurie Santos, "Philosophy—Happiness 5: How Well Can We Predict Our Feelings," Wireless Philosophy, November 9, 2021, YouTube, https://www.youtube.com/watch?v=oB_i5E4fLB4.
6. Christina Armenta, Katherine Jacobs Bao, Sonja Lyubomirsky et al., "Chapter 4—Is Lasting Change Possible? Lessons from the Hedonic Adaptation Prevention Model," in *Stability of Happiness*, eds. Kennon M. Sheldon and Richard E. Lucas (Cambridge, MA: Academic Press, 2014): 57–74, https://www.sciencedirect.com/science/article/abs/pii/B9780124114784000047.
7. Armenta et al., "Is Lasting Change Possible?," 57–74.
8. *Eudaimonic* is derived from the Greek word *eudaimonia*, which is defined as "the condition of human flourishing or of living well. The highest human good." "Eudaimonia," Britannica, last updated September 11, 2023, https://www.britannica.com/topic/eudaimonia
9. Barbara L. Fredrickson, Karen M. Grewen, Kimberly A. Coffey et al., "A Functional Genomic Perspective on Human Well-Being," *PNAS* 110, no. 33 (July 2013): 13684–89, https://www.pnas.org/doi/abs/10.1073/pnas.1305419110.
10. "Positive Psychology Influences Gene Expression in Humans, Scientists Say," Sci.News, August 12, 2013, https://www.sci.news/othersciences/psychology/science-positive-psychology-gene-expression-humans-01305.html.
11. Lauren C. Howe and Kari Leibowitz, "Can a Nice Doctor Make Treatments More Effective?," *New York Times*, January 22, 2019, https://www.nytimes.com/2019/01/22/well/live/can-a-nice-doctor-make-treatments-more-effective.html; Kari A. Leibowitz, Emerson J. Hardebeck, J. Parker Goyer, and Alia J. Crum, "Physician Assurance Reduces Patient Symptoms in US Adults: An Experimental Study," *Journal of General Internal Medicine* 33 (2018): 2051–52, https://link.springer.com/article/10.1007/s11606-018-4627-z.
12. Karen Weintraub, "Growing Tumors in a Dish, Scientists Try to Personalize Pancreatic Cancer Treatment," Stat, October 4, 2019, https://www.statnews.com/2019/10/04/pancreatic-cancer-tumors-in-a-dish/.
13. Luigi Gatto, "Serena Williams: 'I Am a Strong Believer in Visualization,'" Tennis World, April 27, 2019, https://www.tennisworldusa.org/tennis/news/Serena_Williams/69764/serena-williams-i-am-a-strong-believer-in-visualization-/; Carmine Gallo, "3 Daily Habits of Peak Performers, According to Michael Phelps' Coach," Forbes.com, May 24, 2016, https://www.forbes.com/sites/carminegallo/2016/05/24/3-daily-habits-of-peak-performers-according-to-michael-phelps-coach/?sh=79fb95f0102c; Melissa Rohlin, "Phil Jackson and Doc Rivers Use Visualization to Help

Their Players," *Los Angeles Times*, October 9, 2014, https://www.latimes.com/sports/sportsnow/la-sp-sn-doc-rivers-clippers-champions-20141009-story.html.

CHAPTER FOUR: THE SECOND RESET

1. "How Much Time on Average Do You Spend on Your Phone on a Daily Basis?," Statista.com, 2021, https://www.statista.com/statistics/1224510/time-spent-per-day-on-smartphone-us/; Michael Winnick, "Putting a Finger on Our Phone Obsession," dscout.com, https://dscout.com/people-nerds/mobile-touches.
2. Adrian F. Ward, Kristen Duke, Ayelet Gneezy, and Maarten W. Bos, "Brain Drain: The Mere Presence of One's Own Smartphone Reduced Available Cognitive Capacity," *Journal of the Association for Consumer Research* 2, no. 2 (2012): 140–54, https://www.journals.uchicago.edu/doi/full/10.1086/691462.
3. J. Brailovskaia, J. Delveaux, J. John et al., "Finding the 'Sweet Spot' of Smartphone Use: Reduction or Abstinence to Increase Well-Being and Healthy Lifestyle?! An Experimental Intervention Study," *Journal of Experimental Psychology: Applied* 29, no. 1 (2023): 149–61, https://doi.org/10.1037/xap0000430.
4. "Smartphone Texting Linked to Compromised Pedestrian Safety," BMJ.com, March 2, 2020, https://www.bmj.com/company/newsroom/smartphone-texting-linked-to-compromised-pedestrian-safety/.
5. "Too Much Screen Time Could Lead to Popcorn Brain," University of Washington Information School, August 9, 2011, https://ischool.uw.edu/news/2016/12/too-much-screen-time-could-lead-popcorn-brain.
6. Aditi Nerurkar, "The Power of Popcorn Brain," Thrive Global, https://community.thriveglobal.com/the-power-of-popcorn-brain/.
7. Andrew Perrin and Sara Atske, "About Three-in-Ten U.S. Adults Say They Are 'Almost Constantly' Online," Pew Research Center, March 26, 2021, https://www.pewresearch.org/fact-tank/2021/03/26/about-three-in-ten-u-s-adults-say-they-are-almost-constantly-online/.
8. "2016 Global Mobile Consumer Survey: US Edition," Deloitte.com, https://www2.deloitte.com/content/dam/Deloitte/us/Documents/technology-media-telecommunications/us-global-mobile-consumer-survey-2016-executive-summary.pdf.
9. Morten Tromholt, "The Facebook Experiment: Quitting Facebook Leads to Higher Levels of Well-Being," *Cyberpsychology, Behavior, and Social Networking* 19, no. 11 (November 2016): 661–66, https://pubmed.ncbi.nlm.nih.gov/27831756/.
10. Katie Schroeder, "My Grandma Survived WWII. The War in Ukraine Is Making Her Relive Her Trauma," LX News, March 16, 2022, https://www.lx.com/russia-ukraine-crisis/my-grandma-survived-wwii-the-war-in-ukraine-is-making-her-relive-her-trauma/50317/.
11. American Psychological Association, "Stress and Sleep," APA.org, January 1, 2013, https://www.apa.org/news/press/releases/stress/2013/sleep.

12. Jennifer A. Emond, A. James O'Malley, Brian Neelon et al., "Associations Between Daily Screen Time and Sleep in a Racially and Socioeconomically Diverse Sample of US Infants: A Prospective Cohort Study," *BMJ Open* 11 (2021): e044525, https://bmjopen.bmj.com/content/11/6/e044525; Hugues Sampasa-Kanyinga, Jean-Philippe Chaput, Bo-Huei Huang et al., "Bidirectional Associations of Sleep and Discretionary Screen Time in Adults: Longitudinal Analysis of the UK Biobank," *Journal of Sleep Research* 32, no. 2 (April 2023): e13727, https://onlinelibrary.wiley.com/doi/full/10.1111/jsr.13727.
13. "Always Connected: How Smartphones and Social Keep Us Engaged," IDC Research Report, 2013, https://www.nu.nl/files/IDC-Facebook%20Always%20Connected%20(1).pdf.
14. Camila Hirotsu, Sergio Tufik, and Monica Levy Andersen, "Interactions Between Sleep, Stress, and Metabolism: From Physiological to Pathological Conditions," *Sleep Science* 8, no. 3 (November 2015): 143–52, https://www.ncbi.nlm.nih.gov/pmc/articles/PMC4688585/.
15. Andy R. Eugene and Jolanta Masiak, "The Neuroprotective Aspects of Sleep," *MEDtube Science* 3, no. 1 (March 2015): 35, https://www.ncbi.nlm.nih.gov/pmc/articles/PMC4651462/; see also Nina E. Fultz, Giorgio Bonmassar, Kawin Setsompop et al., "Coupled Electrophysiological, Hemodynamic, Cerebrospinal Fluid Oscillations in Human Sleep," *Science* 366, no. 6465 (November 2019): 628–31, https://www.science.org/doi/10.1126/science.aax5440.
16. Pal Alhola and Päivi Polo-Kantola, "Sleep Deprivation: Impact on Cognitive Performance," *Neuropsychiatric Disease and Treatment* 3, no. 5 (2007): 553–67, https://pubmed.ncbi.nlm.nih.gov/19300585/.
17. Ilse M. Verweij, Nico Romeijn, Dirk J. A. Smit et al., "Sleep Deprivation Leads to a Loss of Functional Connectivity in Frontal Brain Regions," *BMC Neuroscience* 15 (2014): 88, https://bmcneurosci.biomedcentral.com/articles/10.1186/1471-2202-15-88.
18. Seung-Schik Yoo, Ninad Gujar, Peter Hu et al., "The Human Emotional Brain Without Sleep: A Prefrontal Amygdala Disconnect," *Current Biology* 17, no. 20 (October 2007): R877–R878, https://www.sciencedirect.com/science/article/pii/S0960982207017836?via%3Dihub.
19. Faith Orchard, Alice M. Gregory, Michael Gradisar, and Shirley Reynolds, "Self-Reported Sleep Patterns and Quality Amongst Adolescents: Cross-Sectional and Prospective Associations with Anxiety and Depression," *Journal of Child Psychology and Psychiatry* 61, no. 10 (October 2020): 1126–37, https://acamh.onlinelibrary.wiley.com/doi/full/10.1111/jcpp.13288; Elizabeth M. Cespedes Feliciano, Mirja Quante, Sheryl L. Rifas-Shiman et al., "Objective Sleep Characteristics and Cardiometabolic Health in Young Adolescents," *Pediatrics* 142, no. 1 (July 2018): e20174085, https://pubmed.ncbi.nlm.nih.gov/29907703/.
20. Séverine Sabia, Aline Dugravot, Damien Léger et al., "Association of Sleep Duration at Age 50, 60, and 70 Years with Risk of Multimorbidity in the

UK: 25-Years Follow-up of the Whitehall II Cohort Study," *PLOS Medicine* 19, no. 10 (2002): e1004109, https://journals.plos.org/plosmedicine/article?id =10.1371/journal.pmed.1004109.
21. Orchard et al., "Self-Reported Sleep Patterns"; "How Does Sleep Affect Your Heart Health?," Centers for Disease Control and Prevention, last reviewed January 4, 2021, https://www.cdc.gov/bloodpressure/sleep.htm.
22. Liqing Li, Chunmei Wu, Yong Gan et al., "Insomnia and the Risk of Depression: A Meta-Analysis of Prospective Cohort Studies," *BMC Psychiatry* 16, no. 1 (November 2016): 375, https://pubmed.ncbi.nlm.nih.gov/27816065/.
23. Jon Johnson, "How Long Is the Ideal Nap?," Medical News Today, October 5, 2019, https://www.medicalnewstoday.com/articles/326803#tips.
24. Rebecca L. Campbell and Ana J. Bridges, "Bedtime Procrastination Mediates the Relation Between Anxiety and Sleep Problems," *Journal of Clinical Psychology* 79, no. 3. (March 2023): 803–17, https://onlinelibrary.wiley.com /doi/10.1002/jclp.23440.
25. Eric W. Dolan, "Bedtime Procrastination Helps Explain the Link Between Anxiety and Sleep Problems," PsyPost.org, October 29, 2022, https://www .psypost.org/2022/10/bedtime-procrastination-helps-explain-the-link -between-anxiety-and-sleep-problems-64181.
26. Maria Godoy and Audrey Nguyen, "Stop Doomscrolling and Get Ready for Bed. Here's How to Reclaim a Good Night's Sleep," National Public Radio, June 16, 2022, https://www.npr.org/2022/06/14/1105122521/stop -revenge-bedtime-procrastination-get-better-sleep.
27. Janosch Deeg, "It Goes by the Name 'Bedtime Procrastination,' and You Can Probably Guess What It Is," ScientificAmerican.com, July 19, 2022, https://www.scientificamerican.com/article/it-goes-by-the-name-bedtime -procrastination-and-you-can-probably-guess-what-it-is/.
28. Floor M. Korese, Sanne Nauts, Bart A. Kamphorst et al., "Bedtime Procrastination: A Behavioral Perspective on Sleep Insufficiency," in *Procrastination, Health, and Well-Being*, ed. Fuschia M. Sirois and Timothy A. Pychyl (Cambridge, MA: Academic Press, 2016), https://doi.org/10.1016/C2014 -0-03741-0.
29. Sun Ju Chung, Hyeyoung An, and Sooyeon Suh, "What Do People Do Before Going to Bed? A Study of Bedtime Procrastination Using Time Use Surveys," *Sleep* 43, no. 4 (April 2020): zsz267, https://doi.org/10.1093/sleep/zsz267.
30. Shahram Nikbakhtian, Angus B. Reed, Bernard Dillon Obika et al., "Accelerometer-Derived Sleep Onset Timing and Cardiovascular Disease Incidence: A UK Biobank Cohort Study," *European Heart Journal–Digital Health* 2, no. 4 (December 2021): 658–66, https://doi.org/10.1093/ehjdh /ztab088; European Society of Cardiology, "Bedtime Linked with Heart Health," ScienceDaily, November 8, 2021, https://www.sciencedaily.com /releases/2021/11/211108193627.htm.
31. Sophia Antipolis, "Bedtime Linked with Heart Health," European Society of Cardiology, November 9, 2021, https://www.escardio.org/The-ESC/Press -Office/Press-releases/Bedtime-linked-with-heart-health.

32. Andrea. N. Goldstein, Stephanie M. Greer, Jared M. Saletin et al., "Tired and Apprehensive: Anxiety Amplifies the Impact of Sleep Loss on Aversive Brain Anticipation," *Journal of Neuroscience* 33, no. 26 (June 2013): 10607–15.
33. Eti Ben Simon, Aubrey Rossi, Allison G. Harvey, and Matthew P. Walker, "Overanxious and Underslept," *Nature Human Behaviour* 4 (2020): 100–10, https://www.nature.com/articles/s41562-019-0754-8.
34. E. B. Simon and M. P. Walker, "Under Slept and Overanxious: The Neural Correlates of Sleep-Loss Induced Anxiety in the Human Brain" (Neuroscience 2018, San Diego, CA, November 4, 2018), https://www.abstractsonline.com/pp8/#!/4649/presentation/38909; Laura Sanders, "Poor Sleep Can Be the Cause of Anxiety, Study Finds," *Washington Post*, November 10, 2018, https://www.washingtonpost.com/national/health-science/poor-sleep-can-be-the-cause-of-anxiety-study-finds/2018/11/09/9180ea10-e366-11e8-ab2c-b31dcd53ca6b_story.html?noredirect=on.
35. Dana G. Smith, "Lack of Sleep Looks the Same as Severe Anxiety in the Brain," *Popular Science*, November 26, 2018, https://www.popsci.com/sleep-deprivation-brain-activity/.
36. "Stressed to the Max? Deep Sleep Can Rewire the Anxious Brain," EurekAlert!, November 4, 2019, https://www.eurekalert.org/news-releases/862776.
37. David Richter, Michael D. Krämer, Nicole K. Y. Tang et al., "Long-Term Effect of Pregnancy and Childbirth on Sleep Satisfaction and Duration of First-Time and Experienced Mothers and Fathers," *Sleep* 42, no. 4 (April 2019): zsz015, https://doi.org/10.1093/sleep/zsz015.
38. Bryce Ward, "Americans Are Choosing to Be Alone. Here's Why We Should Reverse That," *Washington Post*, November 23, 2022, https://www.washingtonpost.com/opinions/2022/11/23/americans-alone-thanksgiving-friends/.
39. "Smartphone Penetration Rate as Share of the Population of the United States from 2010 to 2021," Statista.com, https://www.statista.com/statistics/201183/forecast-of-smartphone-penetration-in-the-us/.
40. Valentina Rotondi, Luca Stanca, and Miriam Tomasuolo, "Connecting Alone: Smartphone Use, Quality of Social Interactions and Well-Being," *Journal of Economic Psychology* 63 (December 2017): 17–26, https://www.sciencedirect.com/science/article/pii/S0167487017302520.
41. "Gallup's 2023 Global Emotions Report," Gallup.com, https://www.gallup.com/analytics/349280/gallup-global-emotions-report.aspx.
42. Vivek H. Murthy, "Our Epidemic of Loneliness and Isolation: The U.S. Surgeon General's Advisory on the Healing Effects of Social Connection and Community," 2023, https://www.hhs.gov/sites/default/files/surgeon-general-social-connection-advisory.pdf.
43. "Loneliness and the Workplace: 2020 U.S. Report," Cigna.com, 2020, https://www.cigna.com/static/www-cigna-com/docs/about-us/newsroom/studies-and-reports/combatting-loneliness/cigna-2020-loneliness-factsheet.pdf.

44. Amy Novotney, "The Risks of Social Isolation," American Psychological Association, May 2019, https://www.apa.org/monitor/2019/05/ce-corner-isolation.
45. Murthy, "Our Epidemic of Loneliness and Isolation."
46. Kassandra I. Alcaraz, Katherine S. Eddens, Jennifer L. Blase et al., "Social Isolation and Mortality in US Black and White Men and Women," *American Journal of Epidemiology* 188, no. 1 (January 2019): 102–9, https://doi.org/10.1093/aje/kwy231; Novotney, "Risks of Social Isolation."
47. "Welcome to the Harvard Study of Adult Development," Harvard Second Generation Study, accessed October 4, 2023, https://www.adultdevelopmentstudy.org/.
48. Tao Jiang, Syamil Yakin, Jennifer Crocker, and Baldwin M. Way, "Perceived Social Support-Giving Moderates the Association Between Social Relationships and Interleukin-6 Levels in Blood," *Brain, Behavior, and Immunity* 100 (February 2022): 25–28, https://doi.org/10.1016/j.bbi.2021.11.002.
49. "Author Talks: Don't Spoil the Fun," McKinsey.com, March 24, 2022, https://www.mckinsey.com/featured-insights/mckinsey-on-books/author-talks-dont-spoil-the-fun.

CHAPTER FIVE: THE THIRD RESET

1. Pierre Philippot, Gaëtane Chapelle, and Sylvie Blairy, "Respiratory Feedback in the Generation of Emotion," *Cognition and Emotion* 16, no. 5 (2002): 605–27, https://doi.org/10.1080/02699930143000392.
2. Bruce Goldman, "Study Shows How Slow Breathing Induces Tranquility," Stanford Medicine, March 30, 2017, https://med.stanford.edu/news/all-news/2017/03/study-discovers-how-slow-breathing-induces-tranquility.html.
3. Susan I. Hopper, Sherrie L. Murray, Lucille R. Ferrara, and Joanne K. Singleton, "Effectiveness of Diaphragmatic Breathing for Reducing Physiological and Psychological Stress in Adults: A Quantitative Systematic Review," *JBI Database of Systematic Reviews and Implementation Reports* 17, no. 9 (September 2019): 1855–76, https://pubmed.ncbi.nlm.nih.gov/31436595/; Xiao Ma, Zi-Qi Yue, Zhu-Qing Gong et al., "The Effect of Diaphragmatic Breathing on Attention, Negative Affect and Stress in Healthy Adults," *Frontiers in Psychology* 8 (2017): 874, https://www.ncbi.nlm.nih.gov/pmc/articles/PMC5455070/.
4. "How to Do the 4-7-8 Breathing Exercise," Cleveland Clinic, September 6, 2022, https://health.clevelandclinic.org/4-7-8-breathing/.
5. Eckhart Tolle, *A New Earth: Awakening to Your Life's Purpose*, 10th anniversary ed. (New York: Penguin Books, 2016), 244.
6. Lin Yang, Chao Cao, Elizabeth D. Kantor et al., "Trends in Sedentary Behavior Among the US Population, 2001–2016," *JAMA* 321, no. 16 (April 2019): 1587–97, https://jamanetwork.com/journals/jama/fullarticle/2731178; Emily N. Ussery, Janet E. Fulton, Deborah A. Galuska et al., "Joint Prevalence of Sitting Time and Leisure-Time Physical Activity Among US Adults,"

JAMA 320, no. 19 (2018): 2036–38, https://jamanetwork.com/journals/jama/fullarticle/2715582.

7. E. G. Wilmot, C. L. Edwardson, F. A. Achana et al., "Sedentary Time in Adults and the Association with Diabetes, Cardiovascular Disease and Death: Systematic Review and Meta-Analysis," *Diabetologia* 55 (2012): 2895–905, https://link.springer.com/article/10.1007/s00125-012-2677-z.
8. Megan Teychenne, Sarah A. Costigan, and Kate Parker, "The Association Between Sedentary Behavior and Risk of Anxiety: A Systematic Review," *BMC Public Health* 15 (2015): 513, https://bmcpublichealth.biomedcentral.com/articles/10.1186/s12889-015-1843-x; Jacob D. Meyer, John O'Connor, Cillian P. McDowell et al., "High Sitting Time Is a Behavioral Risk Factor for Blunted Improvement in Depression Across 8 Weeks of the COVID-19 Pandemic in April–May 2020," *Front Psychiatry* 12 (2021): 741433, https://www.frontiersin.org/articles/10.3389/fpsyt.2021.741433/full.
9. "Sitting More Linked to Increased Feelings of Depression, Anxiety," Iowa State University News Service, November 8, 2021, https://www.news.iastate.edu/news/2021/11/08/sittingdepression.
10. Ben Renner, "Life Gets in the Way: Nearly Half of Americans Want to Exercise, but Don't Have Time," StudyFinds.org, November 23, 2019, https://studyfinds.org/life-gets-in-the-way-nearly-half-of-americans-want-to-exercise-but-dont-have-time/; Debra L. Blackwell and Tainya C. Clarke, "State Variation in Meeting the 2008 Federal Guidelines for Both Aerobic and Muscle-Strengthening Activities Through Leisure-Time Physical Activity Among Adults Aged 18–64: United States, 2010–2015," National Health Statistics Reports, No. 112, June 28, 2018, https://www.cdc.gov/nchs/data/nhsr/nhsr112.pdf.
11. Bethany Barone Gibbs, Marie-France Hivert, Gerald J. Jerome et al., "Physical Activity as a Critical Component of First-Line Treatment for Elevated Blood Pressure or Cholesterol: Who, What, and How?: A Scientific Statement from the American Heart Association," *Hypertension* 78 , no. 2 (August 2021): e26–e37, https://www.ahajournals.org/doi/full/10.1161/HYP.0000000000000196; "The Importance of Exercise When You Have Diabetes," Harvard Health Publishing, Harvard Medical School, August 2, 2023, https://www.health.harvard.edu/staying-healthy/the-importance-of-exercise-when-you-have-diabetes.
12. Glenn A. Gaesser and Siddhartha S. Angadi, "Obesity Treatment: Weight Loss Versus Increasing Fitness and Physical Activity for Reducing Health Risks," *iScience* 24, no. 10 (October 2021): 102995, https://www.cell.com/iscience/fulltext/S2589-0042(21)00963-9.
13. "Exercising to Relax: How Does Exercise Reduce Stress? Surprising Answers to This Question and More," Harvard Health Publishing, Harvard Medical School, July 7, 2020, https://www.health.harvard.edu/staying-healthy/exercising-to-relax.
14. "Exercise, Stress, and the Brain: Paul Thompson PhD," NIBIB gov, July 17, 2013, YouTube, https://www.youtube.com/watch?v=xpy_rAWSWkA.

15. Justin B. Echouffo-Tcheugui, Sarah C. Conner, Jayandra J. Himali et al., "Circulating Cortisol and Cognitive and Structural Brain Measures: The Framingham Heart Study," *Neurology* 91, no. 21 (November 2018): e1961–70, https://n.neurology.org/content/91/21/e1961.
16. "Exercise, Stress, and the Brain: Paul Thompson PhD," NIBIB gov.
17. Hayley Guiney and Liana Machado, "Benefits of Regular Aerobic Exercise for Executive Functioning in Healthy Populations," *Psychonomic Bulletin and Review* 20 (2013): 73–86, https://link.springer.com/article/10.3758/s13423-012-0345-4.
18. Carlo Maria Di Liegro, Gabriella Schiera, Patrizia Proia, and Italia Di Liegro, "Physical Activity and Brain Health," *Genes (Basel)* 10, no. 9 (September 2019): 720, https://www.ncbi.nlm.nih.gov/pmc/articles/PMC6770965/.
19. Ryan S. Falck, Chun L. Hsu, John R. Best et al., "Not Just for Joints: The Associations of Moderate-to-Vigorous Physical Activity and Sedentary Behavior with Brain Cortical Thickness," *Medicine & Science in Sports & Exercise* 52, no. 10 (October 2020): 2217–23, https://pubmed.ncbi.nlm.nih.gov/32936595/.
20. Yu-Chun Chen, Chenyi Chen, Róger Marcelo Martínez et al., "Habitual Physical Activity Mediates the Acute Exercise-Induced Modulation of Anxiety-Related Amygdala Functional Connectivity," *Scientific Reports* 9, no. 1 (December 2019): 19787, https://pubmed.ncbi.nlm.nih.gov/31875047/.
21. Kirk I. Erickson, Michelle W. Voss, Ruchika Shaurya Prakash et al., "Exercise Training Increases Size of Hippocampus and Improves Memory," *PNAS* 108, no. 7 (January 2011): 3017–22, https://doi.org/10.1073/pnas.1015950108; Tzu-Wei Lin, Sheng-Feng Tsai, and Yu-Min Kuo, "Physical Exercise Enhances Neuroplasticity and Delays Alzheimer's Disease," *Brain Plasticity*, December 12, 2018, https://pubmed.ncbi.nlm.nih.gov/30564549/.
22. "Physical Exercise and Dementia," Alzheimer's Society, https://www.alzheimers.org.uk/about-dementia/risk-factors-and-prevention/physical-exercise.
23. Kazuya Suwabe, Kyeongho Byun, Kazuki Hyodo et al., "Rapid Stimulation of Human Dentate Gyrus Function with Acute Mild Exercise," *PNAS* 115, no. 41 (September 2018): 10487–92, https://www.pnas.org/doi/10.1073/pnas.1805668115; M. K. Edwards and P. D. Loprinzi, "Experimental Effects of Brief, Single Bouts of Walking and Meditation on Mood Profile in Young Adults," *Health Promotion Perspectives* 8, no. 3 (July 2018): 171–78.
24. Emmanuel Stamatakis, Matthew N. Ahmadi, Jason M. R. Gill et al., "Association of Wearable Device–Measured Vigorous Intermittent Lifestyle Physical Activity with Mortality," *Nature Medicine* 28 (2022): 2521–29, https://doi.org/10.1038/s41591-022-02100-x.
25. E. A. Palank and E. H. Hargreaves Jr., "The Benefits of Walking the Golf Course," *The Physician and Sportsmedicine*, October 1990, doi: 10.1080/00913847.1990.11710155.

26. Tara Parker-Pope, "To Start a New Habit, Make It Easy," *New York Times*, January 9, 2021, https://www.nytimes.com/2021/01/09/well/mind/healthy-habits.html.
27. Benjamin Gardner, Phillippa Lally, and Jane Wardle, "Making Health Habitual: The Psychology of 'Habit-Formation' and General Practice," *British Journal of General Practice* 62, no. 605 (December 2012): 664–66, https://www.ncbi.nlm.nih.gov/pmc/articles/PMC3505409/.
28. Thomaz F. Bastiaanssen, Sofia Cussotto, Marcus J. Claesson et al., "Gutted! Unraveling the Role of the Microbiome in Major Depressive Disorder," *Harvard Review of Psychiatry* 28, no. 1 (January/February 2020): 26–39, https://doi.org/10.1097/HRP.0000000000000243.
29. Yijing Chen, Jinying Xu, and Yu Chen, "Regulation of Neurotransmitters by the Gut Microbiota and Effects on Cognition in Neurological Disorders," *Nutrients* 13, no. 6 (2021): 2099, https://doi.org/10.3390/nu13062099.
30. Marilia Carabotti, Annunziata Scirocco, Maria Antonietta Maselli, and Carola Sever, "The Gut-Brain Axis: Interactions Between Enteric Microbiota, Central and Enteric Nervous Systems," *Annals of Gastroenterology* 28, no. 2 (April–June 2015): 203–9, https://pubmed.ncbi.nlm.nih.gov/25830558/; Bastiaanssen et al., "Gutted!"
31. Lixia Pei, Hao Geng, Jing Guo et al., "Effect of Acupuncture in Patients with Irritable Bowel Syndrome: A Randomized Controlled Trial," *Mayo Clinic Proceedings* 95, no. 8 (August 2020): 1671–83, https://www.sciencedirect.com/science/article/pii/S0025619620301518; Guan-Qun Chao and Shuo Zhang, "Effectiveness of Acupuncture to Treat Irritable Bowel Syndrome: A Meta-Analysis," *World Journal of Gastroenterology* 20, no. 7 (February 2014): 1871–77, https://www.ncbi.nlm.nih.gov/pmc/articles/PMC3930986/.
32. Daniel P. Alford, Jacqueline S. German, Jeffrey H. Samet et al., "Primary Care Patients with Drug Use Report Chronic Pain and Self-Medicate with Alcohol and Other Drugs," *Journal of General Internal Medicine* 31, no. 5 (May 2016): 486–91, https://www.ncbi.nlm.nih.gov/pmc/articles/PMC4835374/; Rosa M. Crum, Ramin Mojtabai, Samuel Lazareck et al., "A Prospective Assessment of Reports of Drinking to Self-Medicate Mood Symptoms with the Incidence and Persistence of Alcohol Dependence," *JAMA Psychiatry* 70, no. 7 (2013): 718–26, https://jamanetwork.com/journals/jamapsychiatry/fullarticle/1684867; Sarah Turner, Natalie Mota, James Bolton, and Jitender Sareen, "Self-Medication with Alcohol or Drugs for Mood and Anxiety Disorders: A Narrative Review of the Epidemiological Literature," *Depression and Anxiety* 35, no. 9 (September 2018): 851–60, https://www.ncbi.nlm.nih.gov/pmc/articles/PMC6175215/.
33. "The Brain-Gut Connection," Johns Hopkins Medicine, https://www.hopkinsmedicine.org/health/wellness-and-prevention/the-brain-gut-connection.
34. Adam Hadhazy, "Think Twice: How the Gut's 'Second Brain' Influences Mood and Well-Being," *Scientific American*, February 12, 2010, https://www.scientificamerican.com/article/gut-second-brain/.

35. Chen et al., "Regulation of Neurotransmitters."
36. Annelise Madison and Janice K. Kiecolt-Glaser, "Stress, Depression, Diet, and the Gut Microbiota: Human–Bacteria Interactions at the Core of Psychoneuroimmunology and Nutrition," *Current Opinion in Behavioral Sciences* 28 (August 2019): 105–10, https://www.ncbi.nlm.nih.gov/pmc/articles/PMC7213601/.
37. Elizabeth Pennisi, "Meet the Psychobiome: Mounting Evidence That Gut Bacteria Influence the Nervous System Inspires Efforts to Mine the Microbiome for Brain Drugs," Science.org, May 7, 2020, https://www.science.org/content/article/meet-psychobiome-gut-bacteria-may-alter-how-you-think-feel-and-act.
38. Pennisi, "Meet the Psychobiome."
39. Madison and Kiecolt-Glaser, "Stress, Depression, Diet"; J. Douglas Bremner, Kasra Moazzami, Matthew T. Wittbrodt et al., "Diet, Stress and Mental Health," *Nutrients* 12, no. 8 (August 2020): 2428, https://pubmed.ncbi.nlm.nih.gov/32823562/.
40. Eva Selhub, "Nutritional Psychiatry: Your Brain on Food," Harvard Health Publishing, Harvard Medical School, September 18, 2022, https://www.health.harvard.edu/blog/nutritional-psychiatry-your-brain-on-food-201511168626; Giuseppe Grosso, "Nutritional Psychiatry: How Diet Affects Brain Through Gut Microbiota," *Nutrients* 13, no. 4 (April 2021): 1282, https://pubmed.ncbi.nlm.nih.gov/33919680/; Jerome Sarris, Alan C. Logan, Tasnime N. Akbaraly et al., "Nutritional Medicine as Mainstream in Psychiatry," *Lancet Psychiatry* 2, no. 3 (March 2015): 271–74, https://pubmed.ncbi.nlm.nih.gov/26359904/.
41. Chopra, Deepak. *What Are You Hungry For? The Chopra Solution to Permanent Weight Loss, Well-Being and Lightness of the Soul* (New York: Harmony Books, 2013).
42. Cassandra J. Lowe, "Expert Insight: How Exercise Can Curb Your Junk Food Craving: Research Suggests Physical Activity Can Help Promote Better Diet," Western News, Western University, January 4, 2022, https://news.westernu.ca/2022/01/expert-insights-how-exercise-can-curb-your-junk-food-craving/; Shina Leow, Ben Jackson, Jacqueline A. Alderson et al., "A Role for Exercise in Attenuating Unhealthy Food Consumption in Response to Stress," *Nutrients* 10, no. 2 (February 2018): 176, https://pubmed.ncbi.nlm.nih.gov/29415424/.
43. Cassandra J. Lowe, Dimitar Kolev, and Peter A. Hall, "An Exploration of Exercise-Induced Cognitive Enhancement and Transfer Effects to Dietary Self-Control," *Brain and Cognition* 110 (December 2016): 102–11, https://doi.org/10.1016/j.bandc.2016.04.008.
44. Jack F. Hollis, Christina M. Gullion, Victor J. Stevens et al., "Weight Loss During the Intensive Intervention Phase of the Weight-Loss Maintenance Trial," *American Journal of Preventive Medicine* 35, no. 2 (August 2008): 118–26, https://pubmed.ncbi.nlm.nih.gov/18617080/.
45. "Diet Review: Mediterranean Diet," Nutrition Source, Harvard T. H. Chan School of Public Health, last reviewed April 2023, https://www.hsph

.harvard.edu/nutritionsource/healthy-weight/diet-reviews/mediterranean-diet/; Daniela Martini, "Health Benefits of Mediterranean Diet," *Nutrients* 11, no. 8 (2019): 182, https://www.mdpi.com/2072-6643/11/8/1802/htm; Marta Crous-Bou, Teresa T. Fung, Bettina Julin et al., "Mediterranean Diet and Telomere Length in Nurses' Health Study: Population Based Cohort Study," *BMJ* (2014): 349, https://www.bmj.com/content/349/bmj.g6674.

46. Felice N. Jacka, Adrienne O'Neil, Rachelle Opie et al., "A Randomised Controlled Trial of Dietary Improvement for Adults with Major Depression (the 'SMILES' Trial)," *BMC Medicine* 15 (2017): 23, https://doi.org/10.1186/s12916-017-0791-y.
47. Heather M. Francis, Richards J. Stevenson, Jaime R. Chambers et al., "A Brief Diet Intervention Can Reduce Symptoms of Depression in Young Adults—A Randomised Controlled Study," *PLOS One* 14, no. 10 (October 2019): e0222768, https://doi.org/10.1371/journal.pone.0222768.
48. Tarini Shankar Ghosh, Simone Rampelli, Ian B Jeffery et al., "Mediterranean Diet Intervention Alters the Gut Microbiome in Older People Reducing Frailty and Improving Health Status: The NU-AGE 1-Year Dietary Intervention Across Five European Countries," *Gut* 69, no. 7 (2020): 1218–28, https://gut.bmj.com/content/69/7/1218.full.
49. Dorna Davani-Davari, Manica Negahdaripour, Iman Karimzadeh et al., "Prebiotics: Definition, Types, Sources, Mechanisms, and Clinical Applications," *Foods* 8, no. 3 (March 2019): 92, https://www.ncbi.nlm.nih.gov/pmc/articles/PMC6463098/; Natasha K. Leeuwendaal, Catherine Stanton, Paul W. O'Toole, and Tom P. Beresford, "Fermented Foods, Health and the Gut Microbiome," *Nutrients* 14, no. 7 (April 2022): 1527, https://www.ncbi.nlm.nih.gov/pmc/articles/PMC9003261/.
50. Hoda Soltani, Nancy L. Keim, and Kevin D. Laugero, "Diet Quality for Sodium and Vegetables Mediate Effects of Whole Food Diets on 8-Week Changes in Stress Load," *Nutrients* 10, no. 11 (November 2018): 1606, https://pubmed.ncbi.nlm.nih.gov/30388762/.
51. Kirsten Berding, Thomaz F. S. Bastiaanssen, Gerard M. Moloney et al. "Feed Your Microbes to Deal with Stress: A Psychobiotic Diet Impacts Microbial Stability and Perceived Stress in a Healthy Adult Population," *Molecular Psychiatry* 28 (2023): 601–10, https://doi.org/10.1038/s41380-022-01817-y.
52. Katherine D. McManus, "A Practical Guide to the Mediterranean Diet," Harvard Health Publishing, Harvard Medical School, March 22, 2023, https://www.health.harvard.edu/blog/a-practical-guide-to-the-mediterranean-diet-2019032116194.

CHAPTER SIX: THE FOURTH RESET

1. Ann Pietrangelo, "What the Yerkes-Dodson Law Says About Stress and Performance," Healthline, October 22, 2020, https://www.healthline.com/health/yerkes-dodson-law#optimal-arousal-or-anxiety.

2. Kevin Dickinson, "The Yerkes-Dodson Law: This Graph Will Change Your Relationship with Stress," The Learning Curve, Big Think, September 8, 2022, https://bigthink.com/the-learning-curve/eustress/.
3. "Research Proves Your Brain Needs Breaks," Microsoft.com, April 20, 2021, https://www.microsoft.com/en-us/worklab/work-trend-index/brain-research.
4. Marlene Bönstrup, Iñaki Iturrate, Ryan Thompson et al., "A Rapid Form of Offline Consolidation in Skill Learning," *Current Biology* 29, no. 8 (April 2019): 1346–51, https://doi.org/10.1016/j.cub.2019.02.049.
5. "Want to Learn a New Skill? Take Some Short Breaks," National Institute of Neurological Disorders and Stroke, April 12, 2019, https://www.ninds.nih.gov/news-events/press-releases/want-learn-new-skill-take-some-short-breaks.
6. "Want to Learn a New Skill?"
7. "Employee Productivity and Workplace Distraction Statistics," Solitaired.com, September 9, 2021, https://solitaired.com/employee-productivity-statistics; Marriott International, "Americans Multitask More Than Any Other Country—Suppressing Their Creativity and Inspiration," Cision PR Newswire, November 5, 2019, https://www.prnewswire.com/news-releases/americans-multitask-more-than-any-other-country--suppressing-their-creativity-and-inspiration-300951710.html.
8. "Distracted Working," Mopria, https://mopria.org/Documents/Mopria-Distracted-Working-Survey-2021.pdf.
9. Chris Melore, "Multitasking Nightmare: Average Service Industry Workers Juggles [*sic*] 11 Tasks Each Shift," StudyFinds, September 28, 2022, https://studyfinds.org/multitasking-service-industry-workers/.
10. Jason M. Watson and David L. Strayer, "Supertaskers: Profiles in Extraordinary Multitasking Ability," *Psychonomic Bulletin & Review* 17 (August 2010): 479–85, https://link.springer.com/article/10.3758/PBR.17.4.479.
11. Kevin P. Madore and Anthony D. Wagner, "Multicosts of Multitasking," *Cerebrum* 2019 (March–April 2019): cer-04-19, https://www.ncbi.nlm.nih.gov/pmc/articles/PMC7075496/.
12. "Multitasking: Switching Costs—Subtle 'Switching' Costs Cut Efficiency, Raise Risk," American Psychological Association, March 20, 2006, https://www.apa.org/topics/research/multitasking.
13. Kendra Cherry, "How Multitasking Affects Productivity and Brain Health," Verywell Mind, last updated March 1, 2023, https://www.verywellmind.com/multitasking-2795003.
14. Amrita Mandal, "The Pomodoro Technique: An Effective Time Management Tool," National Institute of Child Health and Human Development, May 2020, https://science.nichd.nih.gov/confluence/display/newsletter/2020/05/07/The+Pomodoro+Technique%3A+An+Effective+Time+Management+Tool.
15. M. Csikszentmihalyi, *Flow: The Psychology of Optimal Experience* (New York: Harper Perennial, 1990); Fabienne Aust, Theresa Beneke, Corinna Peifer, and Magdalena Wekenborg, "The Relationship Between Flow Experience and

Burnout Symptoms: A Systematic Review," *International Journal of Environmental Research and Public Health* 19, no. 7 (April 2022): 3865, https://www.ncbi.nlm.nih.gov/pmc/articles/PMC8998023/; Miriam A. Mosing, Ana Butkovic, and Fredrik Ullén, "Can Flow Experiences Be Protective of Work-Related Depressive Symptoms and Burnout? A Genetically Informative Approach," *Journal of Affective Disorders* 226 (January 15, 2018): 6–11, https://doi.org/10.1016/j.jad.2017.09.017.

16. Hannah Thomasy, "How the Brain's Flow State Keeps Us Creative, Focused, and Happy," TheDailyBeast.com, updated June 23, 2022, https://www.thedailybeast.com/how-the-neuroscience-of-the-brains-flow-state-keeps-us-creative-focused-and-happy; Richard Huskey, "Why Does Experiencing 'Flow' Feel So Good?," UC Davis, January 6, 2022, in https://www.ucdavis.edu/curiosity/blog/research-shows-people-who-have-flow-regular-part-their-lives-are-happier-and-less-likely-focus.
17. Ben Clark, Kiron Chatterjee, Adam Martin, and Adrian Davis, "How Commuting Affects Subjective Wellbeing," *Transportation* 47 (December 2020): 2777–805, https://link.springer.com/article/10.1007/s11116-019-09983-9.
18. "State of Remote Work 2021," OwlLabs.com, https://owllabs.com/state-of-remote-work/2021/.
19. Ben Wigert and Jessica White, "The Advantages and Challenges of Hybrid Work," Workplace, Gallup.com, September 14, 2022, https://www.gallup.com/workplace/398135/advantages-challenges-hybrid-work.aspx.
20. "The Future of Work: Productive Anywhere," Accenture.com, May 2021, https://www.accenture.com/_acnmedia/PDF-155/Accenture-Future-Of-Work-Global-Report.pdf#zoom=40.
21. Neha Chaudhary, "Rituals Keep These Athletes Grounded. They Can Help Parents, Too," *New York Times*, July 6, 2020, https://www.nytimes.com/2020/07/06/parenting/rituals-pandemic-kids-athletes.html.
22. Chaudhary, "Rituals Keep These Athletes Grounded. They Can Help Parents, Too."

CHAPTER SEVEN: THE FIFTH RESET

1. Desiree Dickerson, "The Inner Critic," accessed October 4, 2023, https://www.massgeneral.org/assets/mgh/pdf/faculty-development/career-advancement-resources/promotion-cv/theinnercritic.pdf.
2. Michael Bergeisen, "The Neuroscience of Happiness," *Greater Good*, September 22, 2010, https://greatergood.berkeley.edu/article/item/the_neuroscience_of_happiness.
3. Allen Summer, "The Science of Gratitude," Greater Good Science Center at UC Berkeley, John Templeton Foundation, May 2018, https://ggsc.berkeley.edu/images/uploads/GGSC-JTF_White_Paper-Gratitude-FINAL.pdf.
4. Nathan T. Deichert, Micah Prairie Chicken, and Lexus Hodgman, "Appreciation of Others Buffers the Associations of Stressful Life Events with Depressive and Physical Symptoms," *Journal of Happiness Studies* 20, no. 4 (2019): 1071–88, https://link.springer.com/article/10.1007/s10902-018-

9988-9; Erin M. Fekete and Nathan T. Deichert, "A Brief Gratitude Writing Intervention Decreased Stress and Negative Affect During the COVID-19 Pandemic," *Journal of Happiness Studies* 23, no. 6 (2022): 2427–48, https://www.ncbi.nlm.nih.gov/pmc/articles/PMC8867461/.

5. Rick Hanson, "Do Positive Experiences 'Stick to Your Ribs'?" Take in the Good, July 30, 2018, https://www.rickhanson.net/take-in-the-good/; Rick Hanson, Shauna Shapiro, Emma Hutton-Thamm et al., "Learning to Learn from Positive Experiences," *The Journal of Positive Psychology* 18, no. 1 (2023): 142–53, https://www.tandfonline.com/doi/full/10.1080/17439760.2021.2006759; Joshua Brown and Joel Wong, "How Gratitude Changes You and Your Brain," *Greater Good Magazine*, June 6, 2017, https://greatergood.berkeley.edu/article/item/how_gratitude_changes_you_and_your_brain.
6. Hanson et al., "Learning to Learn."
7. Rick Hanson, *Hardwiring Happiness: The New Brain Science of Contentment, Calm, and Confidence* (New York: Harmony Books, 2013), 10, 70.
8. Y. Joel Wong, Jesse Owen, Nicole T. Gabana et al., "Does Gratitude Writing Improve the Mental Health of Psychotherapy Clients? Evidence from a Randomized Controlled Trial," *Psychotherapy Research* 28, no. 2 (2018): 192–202, https://doi.org/10.1080/10503307.2016.1169332.
9. Brown and Wong, "How Gratitude Changes You and Your Brain."
10. "Pandemic Parenting: Examining the Epidemic of Working Parental Burnout and Strategies to Help," Office of the Chief Wellness Officer and College of Nursing, The Ohio State University, May 2022, https://wellness.osu.edu/sites/default/files/documents/2022/05/OCWO_ParentalBurnout_3674200_Report_FINAL.pdf.
11. Charles Mandel, "High Rate of Mental Health Conditions in Women Entrepreneurs 'Alarming,' Reports Flik Study," Betakit, August 30, 2021, https://betakit.com/high-rate-of-mental-health-conditions-in-women-entrepreneurs-alarming-reports-flik-study/#:~:text=More%20than%20half%20of%20women,during%20rounds%20of%20seed%20funding.
12. Pam A. Mueller and Daniel M. Oppenheimer, "The Pen Is Mightier than the Keyboard: Advantages of Longhand Over Laptop Note Taking," *Psychological Science* 25, no. 6 (2014): 1159–68, https://journals.sagepub.com/doi/10.1177/0956797614524581; Keita Umejima, Takuya Ibaraki, Takahiro Yamazaki, and Kuniyoshi L. Sakai, "Paper Notebooks vs. Mobile Devices: Brain Activation Differences During Memory Retrieval," *Frontiers in Behavioral Neuroscience* 15 (2021), March 19, 2021, https://www.frontiersin.org/articles/10.3389/fnbeh.2021.634158/full.
13. James W. Pennebaker and John F. Evans, *Expressive Writing: Words That Heal* (Enumclaw, WA: Idyll Arbor, Inc., 2014); James W. Pennebaker and Sandra K. Beall, "Confronting a Traumatic Event: Toward an Understanding of Inhibition and Disease," *Journal of Abnormal Psychology* 95, no. 3 (1986): 274–81, https://doi.org/10.1037/0021-843X.95.3.274.
14. James W. Pennebaker, "Writing About Emotional Experiences as a Therapeutic Process," *Psychological Science* 8, no. 3 (May 1997): 162–66, https://doi.org/10.1111/j.1467-9280.1997.tb00403.x.

15. Pennebaker, "Writing About Emotional Experiences as a Therapeutic Process."
16. Bronnie Ware, *The Top Five Regrets of the Dying: A Life Transformed by the Dearly Departing* (Carlsbad, CA: Hay House, 2011).
17. Christopher Farrell, "Working Longer May Benefit Your Health," *New York Times*, March 3, 2017, https://www.nytimes.com/2017/03/03/business/retirement/working-longer-may-benefit-your-health.html.
18. Liz Mineo, "Good Genes Are Nice, but Joy Is Better," *Harvard Gazette*, April 11, 2017, https://news.harvard.edu/gazette/story/2017/04/over-nearly-80-years-harvard-study-has-been-showing-how-to-live-a-healthy-and-happy-life/.
19. Julie C. Bowker, Miriam T. Stotsky, and Rebecca G. Etkin, "How BIS/BAS and Psycho-Behavioral Variables Distinguish Between Social Withdrawal Subtypes During Emerging Adulthood," *Personality and Individual Differences* 119 (December 1, 2017): 283–88, https://doi.org/10.1016/j.paid.2017.07.043; Zaria Gorvett, "How Solitude and Isolation Can Affect Your Social Skills," BBC.com, October 23, 2020, https://www.bbc.com/future/article/20201022-how-solitude-and-isolation-can-change-how-you-think.
20. Marta Zaraska, "With Age Comes Happiness: Here's Why," ScientificAmerican.com, November 1, 2015, https://www.scientificamerican.com/article/with-age-comes-happiness-here-s-why/.
21. Attributed to actress Sophia Bush, who posted this quotation on Instagram in 2015.

CHAPTER EIGHT: THE FAST TRACK

1. J. O. Prochaska and C. C. DiClemente, "Stages and Processes of Self-Change of Smoking: Toward an Integrative Model of Change," *Journal of Consulting and Clinical Psychology*, 1983, https://psycnet.apa.org/doi/10.1037/0022-006X.51.3.390; J. O. Prochaska, C. C. DiClemente, and J. C. Norcross, "In Search of How People Change: Applications to Addictive Behaviors," *American Psychologist* 47, no. 9 (1992): 1102–14, https://pubmed.ncbi.nlm.nih.gov/1329589/; Nahrain Raihan and Mark Cogburn, *Stages of Change Theory* (Treasure Island, FL: StatePearls Publishing, 2023), https://www.ncbi.nlm.nih.gov/books/NBK556005/; Lela Moore, "Shifting Behavior with the 'Stages of Change,'" PsychCentral, September 14, 2021, https://psychcentral.com/lib/stages-of-change.
2. "The Hare and the Tortoise," *The Aesop for Children*, https://read.gov/aesop/025.html.
3. Phillippa Lally, Cornelia H. M. van Jaarsveld, Henry W. W. Potts, and Jane Wardle, "How Are Habits Formed: Modelling Habit Formation in the Real World," *European Journal of Social Psychology* 40, no. 5 (October 2010): 998–1009, https://onlinelibrary.wiley.com/doi/abs/10.1002/ejsp.674.
4. Kristin Neff and Christopher Germer, "Self-Compassion and Psychological Well-Being," in *Oxford Handbook of Compassion Science*, ed. E. Seppälaä et al. (Oxford: Oxford Univ. Press, 2017).
5. Jeffrey J. Kim, Stacey L. Parker, James R. Doty et al., "Neurophysiological

and Behavioural Markers of Compassion," *Scientific Reports* 10 (2020): 6789, https://doi.org/10.1038/s41598-020-63846-3.

6. Fernanda B. C. Pires, Shirley S. Lacerda, Joana B. Balardin et al., "Self-Compassion Is Associated with Less Stress and Depression and Greater Attention and Brain Response to Affective Stimuli in Women Managers," *BMC Womens Health* 18, no. 1 (November 2018): 195, https://pubmed.ncbi.nlm.nih.gov/30482193/.
7. Neff and Germer, "Self-Compassion and Psychological Well-Being," 376.
8. Neff and Germer, "Self-Compassion and Psychological Well-Being," 376.
9. Jon Kabat-Zinn, *Mindfulness for Beginners: Reclaiming the Present Moment—and Your Life,* CD (Boulder, CO: Sounds True, 2012).

Index